Focussed Neurology

Focussed Neurology

S Sreenivas MD, DM

Professor of Medicine and
Consultant Neurologist
GSL Medical College
Rajahmundry
Andhra Pradesh

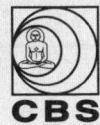

CBS Publishers & Distributors Pvt Ltd

New Delhi • Bengaluru • Chennai • Kochi • Kolkata • Mumbai
Bhubaneswar • Hyderabad • Jharkhand • Nagpur • Patna • Pune • Uttarakhand

Focussed Neurology

ISBN: 978-81-239-2585-1

First Edition: 2015

Reprint: 2018

Published by Satish Kumar Jain and produced by Varun Jain for

CBS Publishers & Distributors Pvt Ltd

4819/XI Prahlad Street, 24 Ansari Road, Daryaganj, New Delhi 110 002, India.
Ph: 23289259, 23266861, 23266867 Website: www.cbspd.com
Fax: 011-23243014   e-mail: delhi@cbspd.com; cbspubs@airtelmail.in.
Corporate Office: 204 FIE, Industrial Area, Patparganj, Delhi 110 092

Ph: 4934 4934   Fax: 4934 4935   e-mail: publishing@cbspd.com; publicity@cbspd.com

Branches

- **Bengaluru:** Seema House 2975, 17th Cross, K.R. Road,
  Banasankari 2nd Stage, Bengaluru 560 070, Karnataka
  Ph: +91-80-26771678/79   Fax: +91-80-26771680   e-mail: bangalore@cbspd.com
- **Chennai:** 7, Subbaraya Street, Shenoy Nagar, Chennai 600 030, Tamil Nadu
  Ph: +91-44-26680620, 26681266   Fax: +91-44-42032115   e-mail: chennai@cbspd.com
- **Kochi:** Ashana House, No. 39/1904, AM Thomas Road, Valanjambalam,
  Ernakulam 682 016, Kochi, Kerala
  Ph: +91-484-4059061-65   Fax: +91-484-4059065   e-mail: kochi@cbspd.com
- **Kolkata:** 6/B, Ground Floor, Rameswar Shaw Road, Kolkata-700 014, West Bengal
  Ph: +91-33-22891126, 22891127, 22891128   e-mail: kolkata@cbspd.com
- **Mumbai:** 83-C, Dr E Moses Road, Worli, Mumbai-400018, Maharashtra
  Ph: +91-22-24902340/41   Fax: +91-22-24902342   e-mail: mumbai@cbspd.com

Representatives

• **Bhubaneswar** 0-9911037372 • **Hyderabad** 0-9885175004 • **Jharkhand** 0-9811541605 • **Nagpur** 0-9021734563
• **Patna** 0-9334159340 • **Pune** 0-9623451994 • **Uttarakhand** 0-9716462459

Printed at: India Binding House, Noida, UP, India

Foreword

I am extremely happy to know that Dr S Sreenivas (neuro-physician) has written a book on neurology.

I have known him for a few years and his teaching, explaining the complex neurology in a simplified manner is amazing.

He has been trained in prestigious medical colleges (deemed universities) which may be one of the reasons for his interest in academics.

He is not only a good doctor, teacher, but also a good orator.

With a lot of information, things become tough and therefore a focussed neurology book would be a great asset.

I wish him all the best in his noble endeavour for trying to encrich the life of many doctors through this exciting book *Focussed Neurology*.

Dr SV Ramana Murthy
Professor and Head
Department of Medicine
GSL Medical College
Rajahmundry, Andhra Pradesh

Preface

The eyes don't see what the brain does not know.

I have always been fascinated by human brain and behaviour. Understanding the functions of brain and its control over the body is both challenging and exciting. 'A thousand miles journey begins with a single step'.

The objective of this book is to present neurology in a focussed manner. The genesis of this book is due to the humble effort I have made in this direction.

I hope you will enjoy reading this book as much as I have enjoyed writing it.

Wishing you a happy reading

S Sreenivas

Acknowledgements

With a deep sense of gratitude I would like to thank

My parents and sisters Mrs S Padmavathi, Mr S Madhava Rao, Mrs S Nagalakshmi and Mrs S Bala Kumari

My brothers-in-law Mr Nagendra Prasad and Mr Hari

My nieces Mrs Neeharika and Miss Kavya

My wife Mrs Phanirmai

My neurology teachers Prof CU Velmurugendran, Prof D Vasudevan, and Prof U Meenakshi Sundaram (Professors of Neurology)

Medical fraternity and management, Shri Ramchandra Medical College and Research Institute (deemed University), Chennai, Tamil nadu

My well-wishers Dr Ganni Bhaskar Rao Garu, Chairman, and faculty, GSL Medical College, Rajahmundry, Andhra Pradesh

My family members, friends and students

Secretarial assistance provided by Dr MB Srinivasa Rao BPT and PGPEC, and Mr A Veera Babu MSc

S Sreenivas

Contents

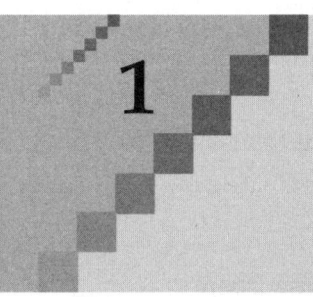

Motor System

1. What is a motor unit?

Ans. The nerve cell, its axons and the muscle fibres they subserve constitutes the motor unit.

2. What is muscle tone?

Ans. The slight resistance that normal relaxed muscles offer to passive movement is muscle tone.

3. What are ramp and ballistic movements?

Ans. *Ramp movements*: Movements that are performed slowly.

Ballistic movements: Movements that are performed rapidly.

4. What is Sherrington's law of reciprocal innervation?

Ans. For a movement to be smooth, the entensor muscles (antagonists) must relax at the same time as the flexors contract.

5. What are the tracts which mediate movement of distal muscles?

Ans. Corticospinal tracts

Rubrospinal tracts.

6. Which tracts mediate proximal limb and axial muscles and help in antigravity postural mechanisms?

Ans. i. Reticulospinal tracts

ii. Vestibulospinal tracts.

7. What is muscle tone and tendon reflex activity dependent on?

Ans. It depends on:
- Muscle spindles and their afferent fibres
- Alpha motor neurons
- Gamma motor neurons.

8. Where does upper motor neuron arise from?

Ans. 40% of fibres arise in the parietal lobe.

60% of fibres arise in the frontal lobe.

9. In what proportion does the corticospinal fibres decussate?

Ans. 80% of the fibres cross.

20% of the fibres descend ipsilaterally.

10. Which body parts have the largest cortical representation?

Ans. The body parts with the most delicate movements have the largest cortical representation.

11. What movements are not affected due to UMN lesions?

Ans. Movements not affected due to UMN lesions are:
- Eyes
- Jaw
- Larynx
- Thorax
- Upper face
- Pharynx
- Neck
- Diaphragms are affected little or not at all.

This happens because these muscles are bilaterally innervated, i.e. stimulation of either the right or left motor cortex results in contraction of these muscles on both sides of the body.

12. Can extra-pyramidal signs occur in internal capsule lesion?

Ans. Yes, because thalamocortical fibres pass through the internal capsule and cerebral white matter. Thus, lesions in these parts affect both corticospinal and extra-pyramidal systems.

13. What is automatisms (synkinesia)?

Ans. It is the activation of paralyzed muscles as parts of certain automatisms. The paralyzed arm may move suddenly during yawning and stretching.

14. What are mirror movements?

Ans. Volitional movements of the paretic limb may evoke imitative (mirror) movements in the normal one or *vice versa.*

15. What are associated movements?

Ans. Attempts by the patient to move the hemiplegic limbs may result in a variety of associated movements. Flexion of the arm and leg may result in involuntary pronation.

16. What is Broadbent's law?

Ans. Lesions above the level of the facial nucleus in the pons affect only the lower part of the face, hand and arm muscles. Upper part of the face and leg muscles are affected only to a lesser extent.

17. What is spinal shock?

Ans. It is a state of acute flaccid paralysis following spinal cord (cervical cord) lesions due to complete acute lesions of the upper motor neurons which not only cause a paralysis of voluntary movement but also abolishes temporarily the spinal reflexes subserved by segments below the lesion.

18. What are the characteristics of spasticity?

Ans. The characteristics of spasticity are:
- Predilection of anti-gravity muscles (flexors of the upper limb and extensors of the lower limb).
- Resistance increases linearly in relation to velocity of stretch.
- Exaggeration of tendon reflexes.

19. What is Babinski sign?

Ans. i. Toe extension when viewed from a physiologic pers-
pective is a flexor protective (nocifensive) response.

ii. A nocifensive flexor synergy involves:

- Flexion of the knee and hip ⎱ triple flexion
- Dorsiflexion of the foot and big toe ⎰ response

20. What is clonus?

Ans. Clonus is a series of rhythmic involuntary muscular
contractions occurring at a rate of 5 to 7 Hz in response to
an abruptly applied and sustained stretch stimulus.

**21. Explain the mechanism and the components of the inverted
supinator reflex.**

Ans. *Mechanism*: It is due to spread of reflexes. The spread being
due to the propogation of the vibration wave from bone to
muscle, stimulating the excitable muscle spindles in its path.
Components: In the case of a lesion of the fifth or sixth cervical
segment, the biceps and brachioradialis reflexes are
abolished and only the triceps and finger flexors whose
reflex arcs are intact respond to a tap over the distal radius.

22. What is abulia?

Ans. Lesions of the frontal lobes have the effect of reducing the
impulse to think, speak and act which is called abulia or
reduced cortical tone.

23. What is apraxia?

Ans. It is a state in which a clear minded patient has no weakness, ataxia or other extra-pyramidal derangement and no
defect of the primary modes of sensation, loss of ability to
execute highly complex and previously learned skills and
gestures.

24. What is ideational apraxia?

Ans. The failure to conceive or formulate an action either spon-
taneously or to command is known as *ideational apraxia*.

25. What is ideomotor apraxia?

Ans. The patient may know and remember the planned action but because the dominant parietal lobe or its connections are interrupted, he cannot actually execute it with either hand, this is known as ideomotor apraxia.

26. What is sympathetic apraxia?

Ans. By destroying the origin of the fibres that connect the left and right motor association cortices, a lesion in the more anterior part of the corpus callosum or the subcortical white matter underlying Broca's area and contiguous frontal cortex on left side causes an apraxia of commanded movements of the left hand, this is known as sympathetic apraxia.

27. What is the commonest apraxia in practice?

Ans. Facio-oral apraxia is the most common in practice. The lesion is left supramarginal gyrus or left motor association cortex.

28. Are dressing apraxia and constructional apraxias really apraxias?

Ans. These abnormalities are not apraxias in the strict sense. They are instead symptoms of contralateral extinction or neglect of the body schema and of extra personal space. They are therefore seen in right parietal lobe.

29. What is diplegia?

Ans. It is a special form of quadriplegia where legs are affected more than arms.

30. What is alien hand?

Ans. i. The hand undertakes complex and seemingly purposeful movements such as reaching into a pocket or handbag.

ii. The patient is aware of the movements but has the sense that the actions are beyond his control.

iii. Infarction in the territory of opposite ACA and left supplementary motor area and corticobasal ganglionic degeneration produces this phenomenon.

31. What is kinetic limb apraxia?

Ans. It involves clumsiness of a limb usually the right or dominant hand in the performance of a skilled act that cannot be accounted for by paresis, ataxia or sensory loss.

32. How does one differentiate between cortical and brain stem lesions of hemiplegia?

Ans. i. *Cortical/subcortical lesion*: It includes presence of
   • Seizures
   • Language disorder (aphasia)
   • Loss of discriminative sensation (asterognosis, impairment of tactile localization)
   • Anosognosia
   • Homonymous visual field defects
   ii. *Brain stem lesion*: It includes ipsilateral cranial nerve palsy with contralateral hemiplegia.

33. What are the common causes of hemiplegia (according to frequency)?

Ans. a. CVA (ischaemia, haemorrhage)
   b. Trauma (brain contusion, epidural and subdural haematoma)
   c. Brain tumour (bleeding into the brain tumour)
   d. Brain abscess
   e. Demyelinative disease
   f. Vascular complications of meningitis and encephalitis
   g. Migraine
   h. Hysteria

34. What are the causes of paraplegia?

Ans. 1. *Acute paraplegia*
   a. Spinal cord trauma (fracture dislocation of the spine)
   b. Haematomyelia (due to vascular malformation)
   c. Arteriovenous malformation of the cord that causes ischaemia by an obscure mechanism
   d. Infarction of the cord
      i. Occlusion of the anterior spinal artery

ii. Occlussion of the segmental branches of the aorta (due to dissecting aneurysm or atheroma, vasculitis and nucleus pulposus embolism)

2. *Less acute paraplegia*
   - Post-infectious myelitis (transverse demyelination)
   - Demyelinating or necrotizing myelopathy
   - Epidural abscess
   - Tumour with spinal cord compression
   - Epidural/subdural haemorrhage
   - Paralytic poliomyelitis
   - Acute Gullain-Barré syndrome

3. *Adult subacute and chronic spinal paraplegia*
   - Multiple sclerosis
   - Tumour
   - Protruded cervical disc and cervical spondylosis
   - Epidural and other infections (tuberculosis, fungal and other granulomatous diseases)
   - Syphilitic meningomyelitis
   - Motor system disease
   - Subacute combined degeneration (vitamin B_{12} deficiency)
   - Syringomyelia
   - Degenerative disease of the lateral and posterior columns of unknown cause

4. *Pediatric paraplegia:*
   - Congenital cerebral disease due to periventricular leukomalacia accounts for a majority of infantile diplegia.
   - Congenital malformation or birth injury of the spinal cord.

5. *Slowly progressive and appearing during childhood and adolescence:*
   - Fredricke's ataxia
   - Familial paraplegia
   - Muscular dystrophy
   - Tumour
   - Chronic varieties of polyneuropathy

35. What are the causes of monoplegia?

Ans. 1. *Monoplegia without muscular atrophy*
  - Cerebrovascular lesion (thrombotic or embolic infarction)
  - Circumscribed tumour or abscess

2. *Atrophic brachial monoplegia*
  - *Infant*: Brachial plexus trauma from birth
  - *Child*: Poliomyelitis or other infection of the spinal cord
  - *Adult*:
    - Poliomyelitis
    - Syringomyelia
    - Amyotrophic lateral sclerosis
    - Brachial plexus lesion

3. *Atrophic crural (leg) monoplegia*
  - Thoracic or lumbar cord lesion
    - Trauma
    - Tumour
    - Myelitis
    - Multiple sclerosis
    - Progressive muscular atrophy
    - Late radiation effect
  - ACA infarction
  - Prolapsed intervertebral disc, retroperitoneal tumour or haematoma.

36. What is Hoover's sign?

Ans. • It is a sign to find out hysterical paralysis.
  • The normal leg fails to demonstrate downward pressure when the hysteric is asked to elevate the supposedly paralyzed one thereby indicating a lack of voluntary effort.

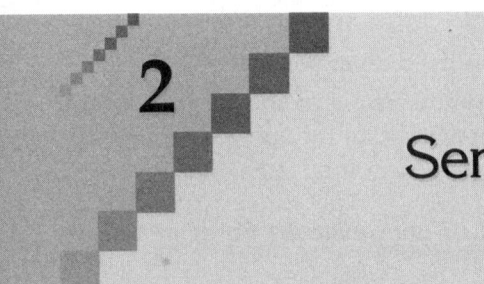

2 Sensory System

1. What is a sensory unit?

Ans. It includes
- The sensory cell in the dorsal root ganglia
- Its central and peripheral extensions, and
- Cutaneous and visceral endings.

2. What are the various receptors for cutaneous sensation?

Ans. Cutaneous receptors respond preferentially, i.e. has a lower threshold to one particular form of sensation.
- Meissner corpuscle .... touch
- Merkel's disc .... pressure
- Ruffini plumes .... warmth and skin stretch
- Krause end bulbs .... cold
- Pacinian corpuscle .... vibration and tickle
- Free branch endings .... pain

3. Classify sensory receptors.

Ans. They are of two types:
1. *Exteroreceptors*:
    - They are present in the skin and mediate superficial sensation.
    - They transduce four types of sensory experience known as sensations or senses. They are warmth, cold, touch, pain.

2. *Proprioceptors*:
   - They are present in the deeper somatic structure.
   - The proprioceptors inform us of the position of our body or parts of our body, of the force, direction and range of movement of the joints.

4. What is the proportion of unmyelinated fibres in sensory nerves?

Ans. In cutaneous nerves, unmyelinated pain and autonomic fibres exceed myelinated fibres by a ratio of 3 or 4:1.

5. What is pallanesthesia?

Ans. Loss of vibratory sense is called pallanesthesia.

6. What is allesthesia? Explain the mechanism.

Ans. A tactile or painful stimulus delivered on the side of hemi-sensory loss is experienced in a corresponding area of the opposite side or at a distant site on the same side. This phenomenon is observed most frequently with right sided putaminal lesion (usually haemorrhage) and with anteriolateral lesions of the cervical spinal cord; it presumably depends on the existence of an uncrossed spinothalamic tract.

7. How do you test deep pressure pain? Give an example.

Ans. *Test*: Lightly pinching or pressing deeply on the tendon muscles or bony prominences.
Example: Tabetic neurosyphylis .... loss of deep pressure pain may be more striking than loss of superficial pain.

8. When is thermal sense confused with pain?

Ans. If the temperature of the test object is below 10°C or above 50°C, sensations of cold or heat become confused with pain.

9. What is tactile agnosia?

Ans. It is a disturbance in which a one sided lesion lying to the post-central gyrus of the dominant parietal lobe results in an inability to recognize an object by touch in both hands.

10. What happens when a peripheral nerve is compressed? When does it become ischaemic?

Ans. *Compression*: It ablates mainly the function of large touch and pressure fibres and leaves the function of small pain, thermal and autonomic fibres intact.
Ischaemia: Ischaemia and procaine have the opposite effect.

11. What is Tinel's sign?

Ans. It is the tingling sensation upon percussion of a regenerating peripheral nerve.

12. What is Phalen's sign?

Ans. Para-esthesia in the territory of the median nerve on wrist flexion is known as Phalen's sign.

13. How do you differentiate parietal from posterior column lesion?

Ans. Vibration sense is lost in posterior column of spinal cord lesions but not in the parietal cortical lesion.

14. What is the characteristic feature of radiculopathy?

Ans. Severe sensory loss in a neuropathic pattern with preserved sensory nerve action potentials indicates a radiculopathy.

15. What are the findings in polyradiculopathy?

Ans. Asymmetrical motor and sensory loss are the features of polyradiculopathy.

16. How does one differentiate between upper medullary and lower medullary lesions?

Ans. i. In the upper medulla, pons and midbrain and the crossed trigeminothalamic and lateral spinothalamic tracts run together; a lesion at these levels cause loss of pain and temperature sense on the opposite half of the face and body.

ii. A characteristic feature of medullary (lower) lesion is the occurrence of a loss of pain and temperature sensation on one side of the face, and opposite side of the body, e.g. Wallenberg's syndrome.

17. **What are the sensory changes due to involvement of sensory ganglia (sensory neuronopathy, ganglionopathy)?**

Ans. *Sensory changes*
  • Unique in that proximal body parts are affected
  • Implicates all sensory modalities
  • Ataxic movements due to involvement of proprioception
  Causes
  • Paraneoplastic
  • Connective tissue disease particularly Sjögren's syndrome
  • Toxic exposure
  • Idiopathic inflammation.

3

Stroke

1. What is Stroke?

Ans. Stroke is a sudden occurrence of a non-convulsive focal neurologic deficit. It is the sudden onset of neurological symptoms caused by cerebral ischaemia or cerebral haemorrhage due to disease of the cerebral blood vessels. Stroke is classified as haemorrhagic or ischaemic and then further sub-divided based on the site of bleed or postulated mechanism of infarction.

2. How common is stroke?

Ans. At least 50% of neurological disorders in a general hospital are due to stroke.

3. What are the three leading causes of death?

Ans. i. Ischaemic heart disease (14%)

  ii. Cerebrovascular disease (9.7%)

  iii. Cancer (5.8%).

4. Discuss transient ischaemic attacks (TIAs).

Ans. i. Transient ischaemic attacks are brief, reversible episodes of focal, non-convulsive ischaemic neurological disturbance, the duration being less than 24 hours.

  ii. Occurrence of carotid TIAs is a predictor not only of cerebral infarction but also of myocardial infarction.

  iii. Vertebrobasilar TIAs are more common than carotid TIAs.

  iv. TIAs cause 20% of infarcts within a month.

5. How frequent are the various categories of stroke?

Ans. Studies suggest that haemorrhagic strokes account for 15–20% and ischaemic strokes for 80–85% of all stroke events.

Of ischaemic strokes, cardioembolism accounts for 15–30%, atherosclerotic infarction accounts for 15-40% and lacunar infarcts account for 15–30%.

Strokes from other causes, such as vasculitis or dissection, usually account for less than 5% of cases.

Up to 30–40% of ischaemic infarcts are considered to be cryptogenic.

6. Classify ischaemic stroke.

Ans. Ischaemic stroke is classified into subgroups based on the postulated mechanism of infarction.

- An embolic stroke occurs when a thrombus from the heart (so called cardioembolic stroke) or another blood vessel (artery-to-artery embolism) breaks away and occludes a more distal cerebral artery.
- Lacunae or small vessel disease develops when lipo-hyalinosis or local atherosclerotic disease leads to occlusion of a penetrating artery deep within the brain parenchyma.
- A stroke is considered to be a haemodynamic infarct when there is evidence of flow failure. Classically, this may involve the border zone areas of the brain (i.e. the regions of the brain at the distal branches of the arterial tree without collateral compensation). This is usually caused by severe stenosis or occlusion of a large artery (e.g. the internal carotid artery).

7. Classify haemorrhagic stroke.

Ans. Haemorrhagic stroke can be subdivided into two types based on the site of the bleed.

- *Subarachnoid haemorrhage*: It occurs when the site of haemorrhage is in the subarachnoid space surroundings the brain. It is usually caused by a ruptured aneurysm.

- *Intracerebral haemorrhage (ICH)*: It occurs when the haemorrhage penetrates into the parenchyma of the brain. It results most commonly from diseases of small blood vessels and amyloid angiopathy (primary ICH) or from vascular malformation (secondary ICH).

8. What is the prognosis in stroke?

Ans. a. 25% of stroke patients recover well.
b. 25% of stroke patients will have moderate disability.
c. 25% of stroke patients will have severe disability.
d. 25% of stroke patients will die.

9. What are the risk factors of stroke?

Ans. a. Modifiable risk factors, e.g. hypertension
b. Non-modifiable risk factors, e.g. age.

10. Discuss hypertension as the risk factor of stroke.

Ans. a. Hypertension is the most important modifiable risk factor for stroke.
b. The risk of stroke (ischaemic and haemorrhagic) is directly related to the degree of hypertension.
c. An increase of 7.5 mmHg doubles the risk of stroke in normotensive patients.
d. The seventh report of the joint National Committee on Prevention, Detection, Evaluation and Treatment of High Blood Pressure (JNC 7 Report) provides guidelines for managing hypertension.

The guidelines emphasize the use of thiazide diuretics alone or in combination with other anti-hypertensives, unless other risk factors indicate the use of different classes of drugs.

11. Discuss diabetes mellitus as a risk factor of stroke.

Ans. a. Diabetes has a direct effect on atherosclerosis of both large and small vessels.
b. Those with diabetes had twice the risk of stroke as compared with those without diabetes, independent of other risk factors.

c. Aggressive treatment of blood pressure among people with type 2 diabetes helps to reduce significantly the risk of stroke by 44%.

12. Discuss lipids as a risk factor of stroke.

Ans. a. Abnormalities of serum lipids (triglyceride, cholesterol), low-density lipoprotein [LDL] and high-density lipoprotein [HDL]) are known risk factors for vascular disease.

b. Cholesterol and LDL have a direct relationship with the incidence of coronary artery disease, while HDL has an inverse relationship.

c. Low HDL and elevated triglycerides have been found to increase stroke risk.

d. Men with a waist-hip ratio greater than 0.93 and women with ratio greater than 0.86 have a higher risk of stroke.

13. Discuss cigarette smoking as a risk factor of stroke.

Ans. a. Cigarette smoking is an independent risk factor for stroke and is still highly prevalent.

b. In studies, a dose-response relationship was apparent. Stroke risk was increased two-fold in heavy smokers (more than 40 cigarettes per day) as compared with light smokers (fewer than 10 cigarettes per day).

c. Even the effects of passive exposure to cigarette smoking have been found to increase the risk of progression of atherosclerosis.

d. The mode of action of cigarette smoking is not entirely clear, but acceleration of atherosclerosis is one possibility. Cigarette smoking was found to be an independent determinant of carotid artery plaque thickness and the strongest predictor of severe extracranial carotid artery atherosclerosis. Other potential biological mechanisms that can induce stroke include:

• Increased blood viscosity
• Hypercoagulability
• Elevated fibrinogen levels
• Enhanced platelet aggregation

- Elevation of blood pressure
- Decreased HDL cholesterol
- Decreased cerebral blood flow.

14. Discuss alcohol as a risk factor of stroke.

Ans. i. The role of alcohol as a risk factor for stroke is controversial.

   ii. Studies have shown an increased risk of haemorrhagic stroke associated with increasing alcohol consumption in a dose dependent fashion.

  iii. Studies have shown a J-shaped relationship between alcohol and ischaemic stroke. There was an elevated stroke risk for heavy alcohol consumption and a protective effect in light-to-moderate drinkers (two or fewer drinks per day) when compared with non-drinkers.

15. Discuss homocysteine as a risk factor of stroke.

Ans. i. During metabolism, homocysteine may be either: Trans-sulphurated to cystathionine, which is converted after further degradation to cysteine or remethylated to methionine.

   ii. The trans-sulphuration pathway is catalysed by the enzymes cystathionine-β-synthase with the cofactor vitamin B_6. The remethylation pathway is catalysed by the 5'-methyltetrahydrofolate-homocysteine methyl-transferase with the cofactors vitamin B_{12} and folate.

  iii. Therefore, decreased levels of vitamin B_6, vitamin B_{12} and folate could cause hyperhomocysteinaemia, which is thought to cause disequilibrium of the coagulation-fibrinolysis status.

  iv. Several studies have shown that hyperhomocysteinaemia is a risk factor for ischaemic vascular diseases including stroke and carotid stenosis as well as microangiopathic changes in subcortical vascular encephalopathy.

16. Discuss carotid stenosis as a risk factor of stroke.

Ans. a. Carotid stenosis is a risk factor for both TIA and stroke.

b. The occurrence of symptoms depends on the severity and progression of the stenosis as well as the adequacy of collateral circulation.

c. In patients with symptomatic disease, the two-year risk of stroke is quite high, approaching 26% among medically treated patients with TIA or minor stroke and an ipsilateral carotid stenosis of 70% or more.

d. For those with asymptomatic carotid artery disease, the annual stroke risk is lower and reported to range between 1 and 3% in those with stenosis of greater than 75%.

e. The prevalence of asymptomatic carotid disease of any degree of stenosis increases with age, occurring in up to 50% of subjects aged 65–94 years.

  • The principal sites for atherosclerotic plaques are the extra- and intracranial large arteries, including the internal carotid artery at the extracranial bifurcation.

  • Atherosclerotic plaques can cause increasing obstruction and artery-to-artery embolism.

17. Discuss transient ischaemic attack as a risk factor of stroke.

Ans. a. TIAs are strong predictors of subsequent stroke. One population based study found a six-month stroke rate of 17% after a TIA.

b. Another study found 10% of patients after TIA had stroke within 90 days and half of those patients had a stroke within two days of the initial TIA.

18. Discuss atrial fibrillation as a risk factor of stroke.

Ans. a. For each advancing decade of age, the incidence of AF nearly doubles.

b. Chronic atrial fibrillation (AF) is a potent risk factor for stroke.

c. The risk of stroke is 20 times greater in patients with AF and valvular disease, and five times greater with non-valvular AF. Even lone AF is associated with an increased risk of stroke.

d. The risk associated with AF is independent of age, hypertension and other cardiac abnormalities.

e. Patients with AF and other comorbidities (older age, congestive heart failure, hypertension, diabetes and prior embolic events) are at even greater risk of stroke.

19. What are the causes of cardioembolic stroke?

Ans. Cardioembolic stroke accounts for 20% of ischaemic stroke.

1. • Non-rheumatic (non-valvular) atrial fibrillation
   • Myocardial infarction
   • Prosthetic valves
   • Rheumatic heart disease
   • Ischaemic cardiomyopathy
2. Warfarin appears beneficial in the prevention of cardio-genic embolism among patients with acute anterior wall myocardial infarction, left atrial or ventricular thrombus and prosthetic valves.

20. What is haemorrhagic transformation?

Ans. If ischaemic damage has occurred to the vascular endo-thelium, subsequent restoration of the blood causes haemorrhage into the infarcted area.

Haemorrhagic transformation occurs in:
• Large infarcts
• If patients are given anti-thrombotic and thrombolytic drugs
• Embolic occlusion when the embolus is lysed by the blood intrinsic thrombolytic mechanism.

21. What are the identifying signs of potential stroke?

Ans.   i. Transient ischaemic attack
   ii. Atrial fibrillation
   iii. Carotid artery stenosis.

22. How does a cerebrovascular lesion present other than ischaemia or haemorrhage?

Ans.   i. Local pressure effects of an aneurysm
   ii. Vascular headache (migraine, hypertension, temporal arteritis)

iii. Multiple small vessel disease with progressive encephalopathy (as in malignant hypertension or cerebral arteritis)

iv. Increased intracranial pressure (hypertensive encephalopathy, venous sinus thrombosis)

v. *Persistent acute hypotension*: Ischaemic necrosis in regions
of brain between vascular territories of cortical vessels
even without vascular occlusion.

23. What causes haemorrhagic transformation?

Ans. Cerebral embolism causes haemorrhagic transformation.

24. Discuss the mechanisms by which strokes arise from atherosclerosis.

Ans. The two mechanisms by which strokes arise from atherosclerosis are:

1. *Artery-to-artery embolism*: Occlusion of the carotid may
   give rise to an embolus that passes distally in the territory
   of the tributary vessels downstream from the internal
   carotid artery.

2. *Watershed or border zone infarct*: Occlusion of the carotid
   artery may lead to ischaemia in the distal field (watershed
   or border zone) in the region of the lowest perfusion
   between its major branch vessels.

25. Which sites correspond to the vascular occlusion?

Ans. i. Headache above the eyebrow ⟶ Carotid artery
occlusion

ii. More lateral at the temple ⟶ Middle cerebral artery

iii. In or behind the eye ⟶ Posterior cerebral occlusion.

26. What are cortical and deep watersheds?

Ans. It implies incomplete compromised blood flow in the carotid
artery.

Cortical watershed: Reducing flow in both the middle and
anterior cerebral territories, the zone of maximal ischemia
lies between the two vascular territories.

• Shoulder and hip weakness

Deep watershed or internal watershed: Lies in the deep portion of the hemisphere between the territories of the lenticulostriate branches and the penetrating vessels from the convexity.

In sufficient haemodynamic compensation, local embolism in slow flow territories may occur. This is frequent in the border zones of the large cerebral arteries (ACA: anterior cerebral artery; MCA: middle cerebral artery; PCA: posterior cerebral artery).

27. What is transient monocular blindness (amaurosis fugax)?

Ans.   i. The internal carotid artery nourishes the optic nerve and retina as well as the brain.

   ii. In about 25% of symptomatic internal carotid diseases, recurrent transient monocular blindness (amaurosis Fugax) warns of the lesion.

   iii. Patients typically describe a horizontal shade that sweeps down or up across the field of vision.

28. How can carotid artery be assessed directly?

Ans. By the presence of bruit (neck vessels) $\longrightarrow$ Low frequencies heard better with the bell of the stethoscope.

29. What does occular bruit imply?

Ans. It indicates more often stenosis of opposite internal carotid artery, sometimes ipsilateral ICA.

30. What are the other signs of carotid occlusion?

Ans.   i. Pulseless arms

   ii. Claudication of jaw muscles.

31. Discuss the vascular anatomy of the brain. What are the typical sites of cerebral aneurysms?

Ans. The brain is supplied by group of vessels known as circle of Willis. The circle of Willis is formed by internal carotid arterial system (anterior circulation) and vertebrobasilar system (posterior circulation).

Typical sites of cerebral aneurysms: 85% occur in the anterior circulation and 15% in the posterior circulation. Three common locations of aneurysms are:
   i. Terminal internal carotid artery
  ii. MCA bifurcation
 iii. Top of the basilar artery.

32. Discuss collateral vessels and modifying effect on cerebral ischaemia.

Ans. 1. *Circle of willis*
   a. Proximal
      i. Posterior communicating artery connects the internal carotid and the posterior cerebral arteries and may provide anastomosis between the carotid and the basilar systems.
     ii. Occassionally, a persistent trigeminal artery connects the internal carotid and basilar arteries proximal to the circle of Willis.
   b. Distal
      i. Over the convexity, the subarachnoid interarterial anastomosis links the anterior, middle and posterior cerebral arteries.
     ii. Capillary anastomotic system between adjacent arterial branches.
2. *Between internal and external carotid arteries*: In occlusion of the internal carotid artery in the neck, there may be anastomotic flow from the external carotid artery through the ophthalmic artery or via the small external internal connections.
3. *Extracranial anastomosis*: With the blockage of the vertebral artery, there is blood flow from the external carotid artery to the vertebral artery via the ascending cervical arteries.

33. Discuss the pathophysiology of cerebral ischaemia.

Ans. 1. *Vascular factors*
      i. Ischaemia begins to appear at 23 ml/100 g/min (normal is 55 ml).
     ii. Infarction begins to appear at 12 ml/100 g/min.

iii. Ischaemic penumbra occurs between 12 and 23 ml/ 100 g/min

iv. Autoregulation occurs between 50 and 150 mmHg.

2. *Metabolic factors*

   i. Excitatory neurotransmitter (glutamate, aspartate) causes increased intracellular influx of sodium and calcium which in turn causes irreversible cell injury.

   ii. High glucose levels in the presence of anoxia causes high lactate which is detrimental.

   iii. A reduction of 3.6°F reduces the metabolic requirement of neurons by 30%.

   iv. *Partial ischaemia*: Brain can survive for 5 to 6 hours or even longer

     Complete ischaemia: Brain can survive for 5 minutes only.

   v. No reflow phenomenon

     Swelling of capillary endothelial cells which prevents the restoration of circulation.

34. What are the ischaemia modifying factors?

Ans. i. Collaterals

   ii. Speed of occlusion

   iii. Blood pressure

   iv. Hypoxia and hypercapnia

   v. Viscosity and osmolality of the blood

   vi. Hyperglycemia

   vii. Anomalies of vascular arrangement

  viii. Existence of previous vascular occlusion.

35. What is autoregulation?

Ans. Constant cerebral blood flow (CBF) is maintained at mean arterial blood pressures between 60 and 120 mmHg, smooth muscle in small arteries responding directly to changes in pressure. CBF is normally independent of perfusion pressure, i.e. there is autoregulation.

In disease, CBF autoregulation can fail. Contributory causes are:

• Severe hypotension with systolic BP < 75 mmHg.

- Severe hypertension with systolic BP > 180 mmHg.
- Increase in blood viscosity, e.g. polycythaemia
- Raised intracranial pressure
- Increase in arterial PCO_2 and/or fall in arterial PO_2.

36. What is ischaemic penumbra?

Ans. i. Following vessel occlusion, the infarct (ischaemic core) is surrounded by an expanding area of poorly perfused tissue (penumbra, oligaemia).

ii. The expanding area of poorly perfused tissue surrounding the infarct which can be salvaged if perfusion is restored within a critical time period is known as ischaemic penumbra.

37. Discuss the cellular mechanisms of stroke.

Ans. The cellular mechanisms in acute cerebral ischaemia are:

Focal cerebral ischaemia inititates a series of events (the ischaemic cascade), which can lead to irreversible neuronal damage and cell death (i.e. infarction) in the part of the brain supplied by that vessel.

The primary effects of ischaemia are:

- Reduced supply of substrate for energy metabolism (oxygen and glucose)
- Reduced removal of lactic acid (acidosis), neurotransmitters and toxic substances involved in the ischaemic cascade
- c. These primary abnormalities can also trigger secondary processes.

38. What are the differentiating points between carotid artery involvement and basilar artery involvement?

Ans. 1. *Carotid artery invo*lvement: Unilateral signs predominate

- Hemiplegia
- Hemianesthesia
- Hemianopia
- Aphasia
- Agnosia

2. *Basilar artery involvment*: Signs are frequently bilateral with cranial nerve, brain stem and cerebellar signs.
   - Quadriparesis
   - Hemiparesis and/or unilateral/bilateral sensory impairment
   - Diplopia
   - Dysarthria
   - Vertigo

39. What is small vessel stroke (lacunar infarction)?

Ans. i. Occlusion of small arteries causing infarcts from 3 mm to 2 cm in the brain.

ii. Small vessel strokes account for 20% of all strokes.

iii. Hypertension and age are the principal risk factors.

40. Describe lacunar syndromes.

Ans. i. Pure motor hemiparesis → Infarction in the posterior limb of the internal capsule.

ii. Pure sensory stroke → Infarction in the ventro-lateral thalamus.

iii. Ataxic hemiparesis → Infarction in the base of the pons.

iv. Dysarthria and clumsy hand syndrome → Infarction in the base of the pons.

v. Pure motor hemiparesis with motor aphasia → Due to thrombotic occlusion of a lenticulostriate branch supplying the genu and anterior limb of the internal capsule.

41. What is Anton's syndrome?

Ans. a. Bilateral infarction in the distal PCA (posterior cerebral artery) produces cortical blindness (blindness with preserved pupillary light reaction). The patient is often unaware of the blindness or may even deny it.

b. If the visual association areas are spared and only the calcarine cortex is involved, the patient may be aware of the visual defects.

c. Bilateral visual association area lesion may result in Balint's syndrome.

42. What is palinopsia?

Ans. Patients may experience persistence of a visual image for several minutes despite gazing at other areas.

43. What is subclavian steal syndrome?

Ans. a. If the subclavian artery is occluded proximal to the origin of the vertebral artery, then there is a reversal of direction of blood flow in the ipsilateral vertebral artery.

b. Exercise of the ipsilateral arm may increase the demand on vertebral flow, producing posterior circulation in TIAs or subclavian steal.

44. What is not a characteristic feature of lateral medullary syndrome due to vertebral artery occlusion?

Ans. Hemiparesis is not a feature of vertebral artery occlusion.

45. What is Binswanger subcortical leukoencephalopathy?

Ans. i. Accumulation of multiple white matter infarcts and lacunae (seen in border zones).

ii. This condition is seen in hypertension and diabetes mellitus.

46. What is the long term prognosis of atherothrombosis?

Ans. i. Among long term survivors, heart disease is a more frequent cause of death than additional stroke.

ii. Pneumonia as a result of faulty swallowing is a major determinant of survival.

iii. If clinical recovery does not begin in 1 or 2 weeks, the outlook is gloomy for both motor and language functions.

47. How are radiological investigations helpful in stroke?

Ans. i. MRI is more sensitive to ischaemic brain damage than CT scan.

ii. CT reveals haemorrhage immediately.

48. What is MRI equivalent of ischaemic penumbra?

Ans. Brain regions showing poor perfusion but no abnormality on diffusion are considered equivalent to the ischaemic penumbra.

49. What is the treatment of atherothrombotic infarction and transient ischaemic attacks?

Ans. i. Management in the acute phase

ii. Measures to restore the circulation and arrest the pathologic process

iii. Physical therapy and rehabilitation

iv. Preventive measures.

50. What is the management in the acute phase of stroke?

Ans. i. Prevention of aspiration and pneumonia

ii. Prevention of venous thrombosis in the legs

iii. Care of the skin, eyes, mouth, bladder and bowel.

51. What are the measures to restore the circulation and arrest the pathologic process?

Ans. 1. Patient to lie horizontal so that circulation to brain is good.

2. *Thrombolytic agents*:
   - 30% of stroke patients treated with thrombolytic agents show complete recovery
   - At the expense of 6% risk of symptomatic haemorrhage (6 to 20% usually)
   - 0.9 mg/kg, 10% bolus, 90% infusion over 1 hour intravenous t-PA

3. Acute surgical revascularisation

4. Treatment of infarctive cerebral edema and raised intracranial pressure
   - Clinical deterioration is worst on the 3rd day

- Intravenous mannitol 1 g/kg then 50 gm every 2nd or 3rd hourly
- Hemicraniectomy
- Surgical decompression for cerebellar infarction

5. *Anti-coagulant drugs*:
   i. *Low molecular weight heparin*:
      - Within the first 48 hr of the onset of symptoms
      - LMWH-4000 units s/c bd
      - Very useful in fluctuating basilar artery thrombosis, impending carotid artery occlusion
   ii. *Warfarin indications*:
      - Severely stenotic cerebral vessel
      - Atrial fibrillation
      - Prosthetic heart valve
      - Certain blood disorders

   Warfarin side effect is haemorrhagic skin necrosis.

6. *Anti-platelet drugs*: Aspirin 325 mg daily.

7. *Symptomatic carotid stenosis*:
   - Surgery and angioplasty for symptomatic carotid stenosis (more than 70% stenosis)
   - *Hyperfusion syndrome*: It develops several days to a week after carotid endarterectomy. The features are headache, focal deficits, seizures, brain edema and cerebral haemorrhage. These are thought to reflect an abrupt loss of autoregulatory ability of the cerebral vasculature in the face of hypertension and increased perfusion in the side of the recently opened artery. Unilateral severe headache is the commonest symptom.

8. *Asymptomatic carotid artery stenosis*: Consider surgery only if the carotid lesion is narrowed to 1.5 mm.

52. What is the role of physical therapy and rehabilitation?

Ans. i. *Plasticity*: Remodeling and reorganization. Restraining that of normal limb forcefully using the sound limb.
   ii. Physiotherapy should be performed within a few days of the abnormal limb.

53. What are the preventive measures?

Ans. a. Aspirin

    b. Anti-hypertensives

    c. Statins

    d. Smoking cessation

    e. Care during surgical procedure.

54. Discuss aspirin.

Ans. 1. Aspirin acetylates platelet cyclo-oxygenase, which irreversibly inhibits the formation in platelets of thromboxane A2, a platelet aggregating and vaso-constricting prostaglandin. The effect is permanent.

    2. Paradoxically aspirin also inhibits the formation in endothelial cells of prostacyclin, an anti-aggregating and vasodilating prostaglandins. The effect is transient.

    3. Aspirin in low dose given once daily inhibits the production of thromboxane A2 in platelets without substantially inhibiting prostacyclin formation. The FDA recommends 50 to 325 mg of aspirin daily for stroke prevention.

55. What is the mechanism of action of clopidogrel and ticlopidine?

Ans. They block the ADP receptor on platelets and thus prevent the cascade resulting in activation of the glycoprotein IIb/IIIa receptor that leads to fibrinogen binding to the platelets and consequent platelet aggregation.

56. Discuss embolic infarction.

Ans. 1. This is the commonest cause of stroke.

    2. 75% of the cardiogenic emboli lodge in the brain.

    3. Patients with chronic atrial fibrillation are about six times more liable to stroke than an aged matched population with normal cardiac rhythm.

    4. Artery-to-artery emboli (source – carotid or vertebral artery)

5. *Paradoxical embolism*: It can occur when an abnormal communication exists between the right and left side of the heart. Thus, embolic material arising in the lower extremities can bypass the pulmonary circulation and reach the cerebral vessels.

6. *Mycotic aneurysm* is a rare complication of septic emboli and may be a source of intracerebral or subarachnoid haemorrhage.

7. *Marantic or non-bacterial thrombotic endocarditis* is associated with lupus erythematosis, cachexia and carcinoma.

8. The point of origin cannot be determined in about 30% of presumed embolic infarctions.

9. In about 30% of cases, cerebral embolism produces a haemorrhagic infarct.

10. *Lone fibrillation*: Atrial fibrillation without other risk factors like diabetes, hypertension, congestive heart failure or cardiac valvular disease.

11. *Haemorrhagic infarct*: Very large infarcts with haemorrhage especially with hypertension. Anti-coagulation therapy should be avoided.

12. *Subacute bacterial endocarditis* which may give rise to embolism has to be treated with antibiotics only.

57. What are the less common causes of occlusive cerebrovascular disease?

Ans. 1. *Fibromuscular dysplasia*: This is a segmental, non-atheromatous, non-inflammatory arterial disease of unknown etiology. Internal carotid artery is involved most frequently with a series of transverse constrictions. There is atherosclerosis in some and arterial dissection in others.

2. *Dissection of the vessels*:
   • Internal carotid artery dissection
      i. Cause is usually traumatic, connective tissue disease
      ii. Seen in women predominantly in late 30s or early 40s
      iii. Relief of pain rapidly with corticosteroids is virtually a diagnostic sign

    iv. MRI shows double lumen, arteriography shows string sign

    v. Treatment with warfarin and heparin till lumen gets diluted by at least 50%

    vi. 85% shows excellent recovery.

- Vertebral artery dissection: Rapid and extended rotational movement of the neck is the most common identifiable cause, e.g. extending the neck to have one's hair washed.

3. *Moyamoya disease*:
   a. Prolonged TIAs characteristically induced by hyper-ventilation or hyperthermia
   b. Parenchymal haemorrhage
   c. Rebuild EEG: A phenomenon in which high voltage slow wave reappears 5 minutes after the end of hyper-ventilation
   d. Seen in young people less than 10 years of age
   e. One part of symptomatology is traced to distal carotid stenosis and another to rupture of the vascular network
   f. Treatment is surgery.

4. *Binswanger's disease*:
   a. It denotes a widespread degeneration of cerebral white matter having a vascular causation and observed in the context of hypertension, atherosclerosis of small blood vessels and multiple strokes.
   b. Dementia, a pseudo-bulbar state and gait disorder alone or in combination are the main features of Binswanger's disease.

5. *CADASIL (cerebral autosommal dominant arteriopathy with subcortical infarct and leukoencephalopathy)*: Similar to Binswanger's disease but without hypertension.

6. *Amyloid angiopathy*:
   - Lobar cerebral haemorrhages in the elderly above 85 years of age
   - Multiple TIAs.

58. What are the causes of stroke in children and young adults?

Ans. 1. Atherosclerotic thrombotic infarction—usually with a recognized risk factor

2. Cardiogenic embolism

3. Non-atherosclerotic vasculopathies—trauma/dissection/SLE/moyamoya

4. Haemotological—sickle cell anemia

5. Hypercoaguable state—postpartum, use of oral contraceptives

6. Inherited deficiencies—anti-phospholipid anti-body syndrome

7. Meningovascular syphilis—exacerbation of inflammatory bowel disease.

59. Correlate oral contraceptives and cerebral infarction.

Ans. a. Hypercoagulability is an important factor in the genesis of contraceptive associated infarction.

b. Cerebral venous thrombosis ⟶ contraception increases the risk 20 fold.

60. What postpartum period is susceptible to stroke?

Ans. Mainly in the 6 week period after delivery.

61. What are the causes of intracranial haemorrhage?

Ans. i. Primary or hypertensive (spontaneous) intracerebral haemorrhage

ii. Ruptured saccular aneurysm

iii. Vascular malformation

iv. Haemorrhage associated with the use of anti-coagulants or thrombolytic agents

v. Cerebrovascular amyloidosis

vi. Bleeding disorders.

62. What are the most common sites of hypertensive intra-parenchymal haemorrhage?

Ans. According to the anatomical distribution of small penetrating arteries arising directly from the main arterial trunks leading to a massive pressure gradient, the hypertensive ICH is often seen in

1. Basal ganglia (putamen, thalamus and adjacent white matter)
2. Cerebellum
3. Pons, but also subcortically in the territory of small penetrating vessels.

63. What is the prognosis of hypertensive haemorrhage?

Ans. Nearly 50% of patients with hypertensive intracerebral haemorrhage die, but others may have a good to complete recovery if they survive the initial haemorrhage.

64. What is Duret haemorrhage?

Ans. The small brain stem haemorrhage secondary to temporal lobe herniation and brain stem compression.

65. What is the CT finding in anti-coagulant induced haemorrhage?

Ans. Before the clot forms, red cells may settle in the dependent parts of the haematoma and forms a meniscus with the plasma above.

66. What are the clinical features of haemorrhage?

Ans. a. Headache
   b. Acute reactive hypertension far exceeding the patient's chronic hypertensive level (because of generalized sympathoadrenal response)
   c. Vomiting
   d. Nuchal rigidity
   e. Seizures
   f. Focal neurologic deficit.

67. Describe hypertensive haemorrhage with ocular signs.

Ans. 1. *Putaminal haemorrhage*: The eyes are deviated opposite to the side of paralysis.
   2. *Thalamic haemorrhage*: Downward deviation of the eyes, pupils may be non-reactive.

3. *Pontine haemorrhage*: Eyeballs are fixed, pupils are tiny but reactive.
4. *Cerebellar haemorrhage*: Eyes are deviated laterally opposite to the lesion, ocular bobbing.

68. What are the poor prognostic signs of cerebral haemorrhage?

Ans. a. Clot more than 60 ml
b. Hydrocephalus.

69. Which anti-hypertensive drugs can be used in stroke?

Ans. 1. Beta-blocking drugs (esmolol, labetalol)
2. ACE inhibitor
3. Diuretics
4. Calcium channel blockers should not be used because intracranial pressure is raised resulting in unfavorable net reduction in cerebral perfusion pressure.

70. What are the conditions for surgical evacuation of hemi-spheric clots?

Ans. a. Lobar and putaminal haemorrhage larger than 3 cm in diameter.
b. Surgical evacuation of cerebellar haematoma 4 cm or larger (because of proximity of mass to brain stem and abrupt progression to coma and respiratory failure).

71. Discuss spontaneous subhyaloid haemorrhage.

Ans. a. Fourth most frequent cerebrovascular disease following atherothrombosis, embolism and primary intracerebral haemorrhage.
b. Those that rupture usually have 10 mm or more.
c. Approximately 90% of aneurysms are on the anterior half of the circle.
They are at
i. Anterior communicating artery
ii. Posterior communicating artery
iii. Middle cerebral artery
iv. Internal carotid artery.

72. Discuss the clinical syndromes of SAH.

Ans. *General features*: Headache, vomiting, few or no lateralizing signs, neck stiffness.

1. *Anterior communicating artery*: Abulia, paraparesis. A collection of blood in anterior inter-hemispheric fissure.
2. *Posterior communicating artery*: Third nerve palsy. A collection of blood in the anterior peri-mesencephalic cistern.
3. *Middle cerebral artery*: Pain behind the eye, hemiparesis or aphasia. A collection of blood in the sylvial fissure.
4. *Internal carotid artery*: Unilateral blindness (at the origin of the ophthalmic artery or at the bifurcation of the internal carotid artery).
5. *Anterior cerebral artery*: Visual field defects.
6. *Cavernous sinus aneurysm*: Sixth nerve palsy.

73. What are sentinel bleeds?

Ans. Aneurysms can undergo small rupture and leaks of blood into the subarachnoid space, so called sentinel bleeds.

74. What is subhyaloid haemorrhage?

Ans. In SAH, blood tracking along the subarachnoid space around the optic nerve is called subhyaloid haemorrhage.

75. What is Xanthochromia?

Ans. Lysis of the red blood cells and subsequent conversion of haemoglobin to bilirubin stains the spinal fluid yellow within 6 to 12 hours of SAH.

76. Which investigations are useful in SAH?

Ans. i. CT head is diagnostic in more than 90%
ii. Angiography
iii. *Lumbar puncture*: Xanthochromia and absence of clearing of blood. Pressure more than 500 mm of water.

77. What is the course and prognosis of SAH?

Ans. a. Patient's state of consciousness at the time of arteriography is the single best index of outcome.

b. Vasospasm and rebleeding are the leading causes of morbidity and mortality in those who survive the initial bleed.

78. What is the non-medical treatment of SAH?

Ans. a. *Surgery*: Clipping
b. *Interventional neuroradiological technique*: Coiling.

79. What is the medical treatment of aneurysm?

Ans. a. Nimodipine 60 mg fourth hourly to prevent vasospasm.
b. Triple H therapy (hypertension, hemodilution, hypervolemia).

80. What are the delayed neurologic deficits of ruptured aneurysm?

Ans. 1. *Rerupture*: 30% within 7 days
2. *Vasospasm*: 30% around 7 days
3. *Hydrocephalus*
4. *Hyponatremia*:
   • Due to inappropriate secretion of vasopressin
   • Secretion of atrial and brain natriuretic factor
5. *Systemic complications associated with immobility*:
   • Chest infection
   • Pulmonary embolism.

81. What is the prognosis in SAH?

Ans. *Immediate mortality*: 30%
Further risk:
• 40% in the first four weeks
• 3% annually later.

82. Discuss arteriovenous malformation.

Ans. 1. An arteriovenous malformation (AVM) consists of a tangle of dilated vessels that form an abnormal communication between the arterial and venous systems usually an arteriovenous fistula.
2. It is a developmental abnormality.

3. The largest ones are most frequently found in the posterior half of the hemisphere (opposite of aneurysm which are located in the anterior circulation).
4. *Clinical features*:
   • Bleeding
   • Seizures
   • Headache
   • Progressive deficit
   • Bruit over the neck, mastoid or eyeballs in young adults is pathognomonic of AVM.
5. *Diagnosis*: Arteriopathy
6. *Treatment*:
   • Surgical excision
   • Endovascular techniques.

83. What are cavernomas?

Ans. Vascular malformations composed mainly of clusters of thin walled veins without important arterial features.

84. What are the two important causes of intracranial bleeding?

Ans. Next to hypertension, anti-coagulant therapy is currently the most common cause of cerebral haemorrhage.

85. What is hypertensive encephalopathy?

Ans. Hypertensive encephalopathy is the term applied to a relatively rapidly evolving syndrome of diffuse cerebral disturbance of severe hypertension in association with headache, nausea and vomiting, visual disturbances, seizures, confusion and coma. The diastolic pressure is above 125 mmHg, grade IV papilledema.

86. What is reversible posterior leukoencephalopathy of hypertensive encephalopathy?

Ans. i. It is due to the accumulation of fluid and has little or no mass effect.
ii. There is bilateral increase in T_2 signal intensity in white matter on MRI and a corresponding reduced density (edema) on CT usually concentrated in the posterior part of the hemisphere.

87. What is eclampsia?

Ans. a. Eclampsia is a form of hypertensive encephalopathy of pregnancy.

b. A safe target is reduction of BP to 150/100 mmHg.

88. What is HELLP syndrome?

Ans. Hemolysis elevated liver enzymes, low platelet count.

89. What radiological investigation is used for arterial dissection?

Ans. MRI with fat saturation is an imaging sequence used to visualize extra- or intra-cranial dissection.

90. Discuss antiphospholipid antibody syndrome.

Ans. 1. Antiphospholipid antibodies (aPLs) are found in a variety of autoimmune disorders, other than systemic lupus erythematosus (SLE) including:

- Rheumatoid arthritis
- Primary Sjögren's syndrome
- Progressive systemic sclerosis
- Takayasu arteritis

2. The method by which aPLs cause thrombosis is unclear. It has been suggested that it may be through inhibition of phospholipid-dependent endogenous anticoagulants, such as antithrombin III, protein C, thrombomobulin or prostacyclin; aPLs could also affect platelet aggregability.

3. The two most frequent tests used to detect aPL are anti-cardiolipin antibodies and lupus anticoagulants.

4. *Sneddon syndrome*: It is associated with
- 32–35 years
- Livedo reticularis
- Livedo racemose

5. *Treatment*: Warfarin, heparin, aspirin.

91. What are the factors which favour venous over arterial thrombosis?

Ans. 1. Slower evolution of the clinical stroke syndrome.

2. The presence of multiple cerebral lesions not in typical arterial territories.

3. Greater epileptogenic and haemorrhagic tendency favour venous over arterial thrombosis.

92. What are the factors that suggest superficial thrombosis of cortical veins and deep cerebral vein thrombosis?

Ans. a. *Superficial thrombosis of cortical veins*
  - Multiple haemorrhagic infarctions without a source of embolism
  - Seizures

  b. *Deep cerebral vein thrombosis*
  - Vein of Galen thrombosis causes bithalamic infarctions.

93. Discuss dural sinus thrombosis.

Ans. 1. *Sagittal or lateral sinus thrombosis*
  a. Sagittal sinus thrombosis
  - Bilateral superficial paramedian parietal or frontal haemorrhagic infarctions.
  - *Empty delta sign*: In the case of CT scan with contrast infusion, a lack of dye opacification in the posterior sagittal sinus can be observed with careful adjustment of the viewing window.
  - Headache, vomiting, papilledema are present.

  b. Transverse sinus thrombosis
  - Temporal lobe convexity is involved.

  2. *Cavernous sinus thrombosis*
  a. Anterior cavernous sinus thrombosis
  - Chemosis, proptosis with 3, 4, 6, V_1 involvement
  b. Posterior cavernous sinus thrombosis
  - No chemosis, 6, 9, 10, 11 (involvement of the inferior petrosal sinus)
  c. Superior petrosal sinus
  - Fifth nerve palsy.

4

Pain

1. What is pain and what are its characteristics?

Ans. i. It is an unpleasant sensation localized to a part of the body.

ii. It has two characteristics:

- *Sensation*: It is perceived by thalamus and hence to somatosensory cortex.
- *Emotion*: It is perceived by thalamus and hence to cingulated gyrus and other areas of frontal lobe.

2. What are positive and negative symptoms in sensory systems?

Ans. Negative symptoms are sensation of numbness.

Positive symptoms are paresthesia and pain.

3. What is balaclava helmet distribution?

Ans. Fibres from back of the face (near the ears) descend up to the spinal cord, whereas fibers from more forward areas descend only a shorter distance in the brain stem and hence brain stem lesions cause a balaclava helmet distribution of sensory loss.

4. What are the two types of pain?

Ans. i. *Nociceptive pain*: Arising from a pathologic process in a body part.

ii. *Neropathic pain*: Caused by dysfunction of the pain perception apparatus itself.

5. What constitutes a peripheral nerve?

Ans. It consists of the axons of three different types of neurons.
- Primary sensory afferent
- Motor neurons
- Sympathetic postganglionic neuron.

6. What are the types of nerve fibres?

Ans. i. A-beta (A-β) ...... Large myelinated ...... responds to light touch.

ii. A-delta (A-δ) and C ...... Less myelinated ...... responds to intense painful stimuli.

7. What is sensitization?

Ans. In a sensitized tissue, normally innocuous stimuli can produce pain, e.g. sunburned skin.

8. What is substance P?

Ans. It plays a vital role in the mechanism of pain.

i. It causes vasodilation and neurogenic oedema with further accumulation of bradykinin.

ii. It also releases histamine (H) from mast cells and serotonin (5 HT) from platelets.

9. What is referred pain?

Ans. The spatial displacement of pain sensation from the site of injury that produces is known as referred pain.

10. What is neuropathic pain?

Ans. It is due to:
- Increased sensitivity.
- Spontaneous activity (begins to generate impulses in the absence of stimulation) is due to an increased concentration of sodium channels.

11. What is sympathetically mediated pain?

Ans. i. This implies that sympathetic activity can activate undamaged nociceptors when inflammation is present.

ii. Signs of sympathetic hyperactivity should be sought in patients with post-traumatic pain and inflammation and no other obvious explanation.

12. What are COX-1 and COX-2 inhibitors?

Ans.   i. COX-1 inhibitors are constitutively expressed.
COX-2 inhibitors are induced in inflammatory state.
ii. COX inhibitors does not impair platelet mediated mechanism.

13. What is dysesthesia?

Ans. Any abnormal sensation described as unpleasant by the patient is known as dysesthesia.

14. What is paresthesia?

Ans. Mainly spontaneous abnormal sensation that is not unpleasant usually described as paresthesia.

15. What is allodynia?

Ans. Abnormal perception of pain from a normally non-painful mechanical or thermal stimulus usually has elements of delay in perception or of after sensation.

16. What is skin pain?

Ans. Skin pain is of two types:
• Pricking (*fast*) pain: The first pain is thought to be transmitted by the larger (A, δ) fibres
• Stinging or burning pain (*slow*): The second pain is transmitted by the thinner unmyelinated C-fibres which is somewhat more diffused and longlasting.

17. What are endogenous pain control activators?

Ans.   i. Prolonged pain
ii. Fear is the most powerful activator of this endogenous opioid mediated modulating system.

18. What is Walter Cannon's law of denervation supersensitivity?

Ans. When a group of neurons is deprived of its natural innervations, they become hyperactive.

19. How are sodium channel blockers useful as treatment for neurogenic pain?

Ans. Sodium channels accumulate at the site of a neuroma and all along the axon after nerve injury which gives rise to ectopic and spontaneous activity of the sensory nerve cell and axon.

This mechanism is concordant with the relief of neurogenic pain by sodium-channel blocking anti-convulsants.

20. How are trycyclic anti-depressants useful in the control of pain?

Ans. They block serotonin reuptake and facilitate the action of the intrinsic opiate analgesic system.

21. What is causalgia?

Ans. It is persistent burning pain and abnormalities of sympathetic innervations consequent upon trauma to a major nerve in an extremity.

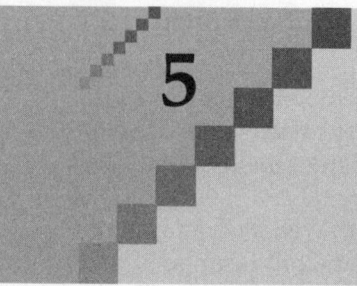

Headache

1. What are the characteristic features of migraine?

Ans. There are three characteristic features which are:
- Paroxysmal headache
- Nausea/vomiting
- Aura of focal neurological events (usually visual)
  - *Classic migraine*: It has all the three features.
  - *Common migraine*: Paroxysmal headache is present. Vomiting may or may not be present. Aura is not present.

2. What is complicated migraine?

Ans. In a small number of patients, the symptoms of aura do not resolve leaving more permanent neurological disturbance.

3. What is migraine equivalent?

Ans. In some patients, the focal events may occur by themselves without headache.

4. What is the characteristic feature of headache due to raised intracranial tension (ICT)?

Ans. The headache of raised ICT is present on waking and often resolves or improves as the patient becomes upright (reducing the intracranial pressure) or takes simple analgesics.

5. What is tension type headache?

Ans. Headache that persists for weeks, present all day and poorly responsive to simple analgesics is very likely to be tension type headache, whatever their other characteristics. In contrast to migraine, there is no associated vomiting or photophobia.

6. What is insignificant headache?

Ans. Headache so well localized by the patient that a finger is used to locate the exact spot on the skull are never associated with significant disease.

7. Correlate headache with local tenderness.

Ans. 1. *Trigeminal neuralgia*: Acute pain precipitated by skin contact.
2. *Temporal arteritis*: Exquisite tenderness.

8. What are the dietary agents which precipitate headache?

Ans. • Cheese
• Chocolate
• Red wine.

9. What is SUNCT?

Ans. Shortlasting unilateral neuralgiform headache with conjunctival injection and tearing. Treatment is with indomethacin.

10. What are the characteristics of facial pain?

Ans. Trigeminal neuralgia ...... 2nd and 3rd divisions of 5th nerve get affected.
Postherpetic neuralgia ...... 1st division of 5th nerve gets affected.

11. What is the mechanism of trigeminal neuralgia?

Ans. Compression of the trigeminal nerve rootlets at their entry to the brain stem by aberrant loops of the cerebellar arteries.

12. What is the mechanism of migraine?

Ans. *Vascular theory of migraine*: Headache phase of migraine attacks are caused by extracranial vasodilatation and the neurologic symptoms are produced by intracranial vasoconstriction.

Neuronal theory of migraine: The dorsal raphe cells stop firing during deep sleep is known to ameliorate migraine. The anti-migraine prophylactic drugs also inhibit activity of the dorsal raphe cells through a direct or indirect agonist effect.

13. What is the relationship of stress and migraine?

Ans. Patients with migraine do not encounter more stress than headache free individuals, over-responsiveness to stress appears to be the issue.

14. What induces dental pain?

Ans. A cold stimulus will repeatedly induce dental pain.

15. Correlate pain with provocating factors.

Ans.   i. *During chewing*:

      a. Trigeminal neuralgia

      b. Temporomandibular joint dysfunction

      c. Giant cell arteritis (jaw claudication).

  ii. *Swallowing and taste provocation*:

      a. Glossopharyngeal neuralgia.

16. What are the conditions associated with headache and hypertension?

Ans. Phaeochromocytoma and malignant hypertension are the two exceptions to the generalization that hypertension per se is a very uncommon cause of headache. Diastolic pressure of at least 120 mmHg are requisite for hypertension to cause headache.

17. What is the treatment for cough headache?

Ans. Treatment is indomethacin 50 to 200 mg daily.

18. What is the cause of post lumbar-puncture headache?

Ans. Loss of CSF volume decreases the brain's supporting cushion so that when a patient is upright, there is probably dilatation and tension placed on the brain's anchoring structure, the pain sensitive dural sinuses resulting in pain.

19. What are triptans?

Ans. The triptans are potent agonists of 5-HT1B, 5-HT1D and 5-HT1E and only 5-HT1B efficacy is currently thought to be essential for anti-migraine therapy.

20. What is the relationship of migraine with dopamine?

Ans. Most migraine symptoms are induced by dopaminergic stimulation.

21. What is empty neuron theory of migraine?

Ans. Norepinephrine alleviates migraine, therefore migraine susceptibility may relate to genetically based variations in the ability to maintain adequate concentration of certain neurotransmitters within postganglionic sympathetic nerve terminals. This hypothesis has been called the empty neuron theory of migraine.

22. What is the treatment of migraine?

Ans. i. Anti-inflammatory agents

ii. 5HT1—agonists

iii. Dopamine antagonists.

23. What is the IV protocol for migraine?

Ans. Administration over 2 minutes of a mixture of 5 mg of prochlorperazine and 0.5 mg of dihydroergotamine.

24. What is the prophylactic treatment of migraine?

Ans. Once effective stabilization is achieved, the drug is continued for 5 to 6 months and then tapered to assess the continued need.

25. What is the pathognomonic feature of cluster headache?

Ans. *Pathognomonic feature*: Alcohol provokes attacks in about 70% of patients but ceases to be provocative when bout remits, this on-off vulnerability to alcohol is pathognomonic of cluster headache.

26. What is the prophylaxis and treatment of cluster headache?

Ans. 1. *Prophylaxis*
   a. Lithium 600 to 900 mg daily
   b. Prednisolone 60 mg for 7 days.
2. *Treatment*
   a. Inhalation of 100% oxygen for 10 to 15 minutes at the onset of headache may also abort the attack.
   b. Sumatriptan 6 mg subcutaneously.

27. What are the disorders of headache which have benign and grave implications?

Ans. 1. Migraine
2. Cluster headache   } Benign implications
3. Tic douloureux
4. Meningitis   } Grave implications
5. Subarachnoid haemorrhage

28. What are the pain sensitive cranial structures?

Ans. i. Skin, subcutaneous, muscles, extracranial arteries and periosteum of the skull.
  ii. Delicate structures of the eye, ear, nasal cavities and paranasal sinuses.
 iii. Intracranial venous sinuses and their large tributaries especially pericavernous structures.
 iv. Parts of the dura at the base of the brain and the arteries within the dura and pia-arachnoid particularly the proximal parts of the anterior and middle cerebral arteries and the intracranial segment of the internal carotid artery.
  v. Middle meningeal and superficial temporal arteries.
 vi. Optic, oculomotor, trigeminal, glossopharyngeal and first three cranial nerves.

29. Where is the pain referred to—from supratentorial and infra-tentorial regions?

Ans. *Pain from supratentorial region*: To the anterior 2/3rd of the head via 1st and 2nd divisions of 5th nerve.

Pain from infratentorial regions: To the vertex and back of the head and neck via upper cervical roots.

30. What are the mechanisms of cranial pain?

Ans. 1. *Dilatation of intracranial or extracranial arteries*: Increased pulsation of meningeal vessels activates pain – sensitive structures within their walls or around the base of the brain

2. *Activation of the trigeminovascular system*: The trigeminal nerves and the blood vessels they supply.

3. Infection or blockage of the paranasal sinuses

4. Headache of ocular origin

5. Headache that accompany diseases of ligaments, muscles and apophyseal joints in the upper part of the cervical spine

6. Headache of meningeal irritation

7. Lumbar puncture headache

8. *Headaches that are aggravated by lying down*:
   a. Subdural haematomas and brain tumours particularly those in the posterior fossa.
   b. In all these states of raised intracranial pressure, headaches are typically aggravated in the early morning after a long period of recumbency.

9. Exertional headaches.

31. What is the relationship of 80% and migraine?

Ans. 1. It is seen in successive generations in 80% of cases.

2. In more than 80% of patients, the onset is before 30 years of age.

32. What are migraine variants?

Ans. 1. *Basilar migraine*

2. *Hemiplegic migraine*

3. *Complicated migraine*: Rarely neurologic symptoms instead of being transitory. May leave a permanent deficit (homonymous visual field defects) indicative of an ischaemic stroke.

33. What is status migrainous?

Ans. i. Migraine that lapses into a condition of daily or virtually severe continuous headache.

ii. *Treatment*: Administer corticosteroids, one of the triptan medications or ergots intravenously in selected patients.

iii. Metoclopramide 10 mg IV followed by DHE 0.5 to 1 mg IV 8th hourly for 2 days.

34. What is the pathogenesis of migraine?

Ans. i. Trigeminal vascular reflex which releases vasogenic substances into the vessel walls is the most plausible explanation of the headache.

ii. Spreading depression as the best explanation of the neurologic deficit.

35. What is indomethacin–responsive headache?

Ans. Headaches responsive to indomethacin are:
- Orgasmic headache
- Premenstrual and perimenstrual migraine
- Chronic paroxysmal hemicrania
- Exertional headache.

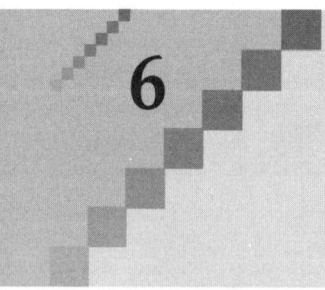

6

Backache and Neck Pain

1. What are the general clinical features of low back pain?

Ans. The features are:

i. *Pain*: It may be
- local
- referred
- radicular
- arising from secondary (protective) muscular spasms

ii. *Stiffness*

iii. *Limitation of movement*

iv. *Deformity.*

2. What is gibbus?

Ans. A sharp kyphotic angulation usually indicative of a fracture is gibbus.

3. What is trendelenburg sign?

Ans. Pelvic tilt or obliquity is trendelenburg sign.

4. What is the normal extent of straight leg raising (SLR)?

Ans. Passive SLR is possible up to 90° in normal individuals.

5. What is Lasègue's sign?

Ans. In diseases of a lumbosacral joints and roots, passive SLR evokes pain and is restricted to the affected side. This is known as Lasègue's sign.

6. What is crossed SLR?

Ans. The crossed SLR is less sensitive but more specific for disc herniation than the SLR sign. The nerve or nerve root lesion is always on the side of the pain.

7. What is reverse SLR sign?

Ans. i. In this, hyperextension of the spine is most limited and reproduces pain.

ii. This maneuver which stretches L2-4 nerve roots and the femoral nerve is considered positive if the patient's usual back or limb pain is reproduced.

8. What is Patrick's test?

Ans. a. It is a helpful indicator of hip disease.

b. With the patient's supine, the heel of the offending leg is placed on the opposite knee and pain is evoked by depressing the flexed leg and externally rotating the hip.

9. What is Spurling's sign?

Ans. Extension and lateral rotation of the neck narrows the intervertebral foramen and may produce radicular symptoms. This is known as Spurling's sign.

10. What is Lhermitte's symptom?

Ans. a. It may be present in cervical spondylosis.

b. An electric sensation elicited by neck flexion and radiating pain down the spine from the neck usually indicates involvement of the cervical or upper thoracic (T_1–T_2) spine.

11. What are the differentiating points of pain between (i) Lumbar disc disease, (ii) Vascular claudication and (iii) Lumbar canal stenosis?

Ans. i. *Lumbar disc disease*: Pain is produced by sitting. Sitting stretches the sciatic nerve (L_5 and S_1 roots) because the nerve passes posterior to the hip.

ii. *Vascular claudication*: Pain is provoked by walking.

iii. *Lumbar canal stenosis*: Symptoms are often provoked by standing and are relieved by sitting.

12. What does tenderness over a spinous process indicate?

Ans. i. Presence of inflammation (disc space infection)

ii. Pathologic fracture

iii. Spinal metastasis

iv. Disc lesion at the site deep to it.

13. What is spondylolysis?

Ans. It consists of a bony defect in the pars interarticularis (the segment at the junction of the pedicle and lamina).

14. What is the characteristic feature of strain?

Ans. It is characteristically worsened by abduction of the thigh against resistance and is also felt in the symphysis pubis or groin.

15. How does one differentiate between L_5 root and S_1 root?

Ans. L_5 root:

- It causes weakness of dorsiflexion.
- Therefore, there is difficulty in walking on heels.
- Causes foot drop.

S_1 root:

- It causes weakness of plantar flexion.
- Therefore, it causes difficulty in walking on toes.
- Ankle jerk is lost.

16. What is disc bulge? Also define disc protrusion and disc extrusion.

Ans. i. *Disc bulge (50%):* Symmetrical expansion of the disc beyond the margins of the interspace.

ii. *Disc protrusion (25%):* Asymmetrical extension of the disc beyond the interspace.

iii. *Disc extrusion (1%):* More extreme extension of the disc.

17. What is the conservative treatment of ruptured lumbar disc?

Ans. i. Oral dexamethasone for several days 4 mg every 8th hourly.

ii. Protection of brace or light spinal support.

iii. Traction is of little use in lumbar disc disease.

18. What is the indication of surgery in ruptured lumbar disc?

Ans. a. The only indication for emergency surgery is an acute compression of the cauda equina by massive disc extrusion causing

- bilateral sensorimotor loss and sphincteric paralysis.
- severe unilateral motor loss.

b. The surgical procedure most often indicated for lumbar disc disease is a hemilaminectomy with excision of disc fragments.

19. How does one differentiate between neoplastic and infectious diseases of the spine?

Ans. i. *Infection*: Disc space is involved.

ii. *Cancer*: Disc space is not involved.

20. What is the important cause of backache from visceral disease?

Ans. The uterosacral ligaments is the most important pelvic source of chronic back pain.

21. What are the preventive aspects of lower back pain?

Ans. a. One should always lift objects close to the body.

b. Sudden strenuous activity without conditioning and warm-up is likely to injure disease and ligamentous envelope.

22. What happens to sensory nerve conduction studies when nerve root is damaged?

Ans. They are normal when focal sensory loss is due to nerve root damage because the nerve roots are proximal to the nerve cell bodies in the dorsal root ganglia.

23. What is the characteristic feature of ankylosing spondylitis?

Ans. a. Back pain improving with exercise is characteristic.

b. Onset is at a young age.

24. What are the three categories for pain in the neck?

Ans. The three categories of painful disease in the neck are:
i. Cervical spine
ii. Brachial plexus
iii. Shoulder.

25. What is thoracic outlet syndrome?

Ans. The combination of:
i. Circulatory abnormalities
ii. Signs referable to the medial cord of the brachial plexus is characteristic of thoracic outlet syndrome.

26. When does spinal canal narrowing produce symptoms?

Ans. The spinal canal narrowing to less than 10 to 11 cm in the anteroposterior diameter produces symptoms.

27. What is the radiological investigation which is useful in atlantoaxial dislocation?

Ans. Cautiously performed lateral radiographs in flexion and extension are useful in visualizing atlantoaxial dislocation or subluxation of the lower segments.

28. What are the roots commonly involved in cervical disc herniation?

Ans. The roots most commonly involved are:
- 7th (70%)
- 6th (20%).

29. What are the treatment modalities of cervical disc herniation?

Ans. • *Medical treatment*: 2 to 10 lb of upward traction is useful.
• *Surgical treatment*: Anterior approach is useful.

30. What are the features of thoracic outlet syndrome?

Ans. i. Anatomic anomalies in the lateral cervical region compresses
- Brachial plexus
- Subclavian artery
- Subclavian vein

   ii. Female to male ratio 5:1 due to:
   * Sagging of the shoulder
   * Large breasts
   * Poor muscular tone
   iii. An anomalous cervical rib which arises from 7th cervical vertebra is the commonest cause.

31. What is Adson's test?

Ans. It is the conventional test for compression of the subclavian artery. With extension of the neck and turning of the chin to the affected side, the tension on the anterior scalene muscle is increased and the subclavian artery compressed resulting in a supraclavicular bruit and obliteration of the radial pulse.

7
Speech Disorders and Cortical Functions

1. What is language?

Ans. Language allows the communication and elaboration of thoughts and experiences by linking them to arbitrary symbols known as words.

2. What is speech?

Ans. Speech is the process whereby vocal sounds are used to convey meaning between individuals.

3. On which side is the speech centre situated?

Ans. In approximately 90% of right handers and 60% of the left handers, the speech centre is situated on the left side.

4. What is crossed aphasia?

Ans. A language disturbance occurring after a right hemispheric lesion in a right hander is known as crossed aphaxia.

5. What is anomia?

Ans. Anomia is a deficit of naming. It is the single most common finding in aphasic patients.

6. Does the non-dominant lobe have any role in speech? What is prosody?

Ans. Yes, the non-dominant parietal lobe controls the non-verbal aspects of speech and intonation.

Prosody (intonation and stress) is present in right hemisphere.

7. What is a characteristic feature of transcortical aphasia?

Ans. The characteristic feature of transcortical aphasia is repetition being spared.

Repetition is affected by lesions around sylvian fissure and therefore in transcortical aphasia where sylvian fissure is not affected, repetition is spared.

8. What is association cortex?

Ans. It is the cortex with no definite specialized area. It has a less specialized area.

9. What is paraphasia?

Ans. Paraphasia indicates wrong word.

There are two types of paraphasia:
1. *Semantic paraphasia*: It is an incorrect but legitimate word, e.g. pen for pencil.
2. *Phonemic paraphasia*: It is phonetically inaccurate, e.g. plentil for pencil.

10. What is non-fluent speech?

Ans. Average utterance length is below four words.

11. What is alexia?

Ans. Alexia is an inability to either read aloud or comprehend single words and simple sentences.

12. What is agraphia or dysgraphia?

Ans. It is used to describe an acquired deficit in the spelling or grammar of written language.

13. What is anosognosia?

Ans. Some patients with negligence may deny the existence of hemiparesis and may also deny ownership of the paralyzed limb, this condition is known as anosognosia.

14. What is diaschisis?

Ans. Diaschisis means remote dysfunction.
  • Some parts of the initial deficits appear to arise from remote dysfunction (diaschisis) in parts of the brain that are interconnected with the site of initial injury.

- Improvement in these patients may reflect at least in part a normalization of the remote dysfunction.

15. What are the two epicenters of the language network, the disorders of which cause central syndrome?

Ans. The two epicenters of the language network are Broca's and Wernicke's areas, the disorders of which cause central syndrome.

16. What are subcortical aphasias?

Ans. Aphasia due to involvement of subcortical structures like:
- Striatum
- Thalamus of the left hemisphere.

They may present with combinations like:
- Fluent aphasia with hemiparesis
- Anomic aphasia accompanied by dysarthria.

17. What is aphemia (pure word mutism)?

Ans.
- It is acute onset of severely impaired fluency (often mutism). It causes the patient to be wordless (mute) but leaves inner speech intact and writing undisturbed.
- It is due to partial lesions of Broca's area.
- Recovery is the rule (transience).

18. What is the central language area?

Ans. Perisylvian region is the central language area.

19. What are the components of comprehension?

Ans.
- *Perception of spoken and internal language*: Wernicke's area (22, 41, 42).
- *Perception of written language*: Angular Gyrus (39).

20. What are the components of executive or output region?

Ans.
- *Motor aspects of speech*: Broca's area (44, 45).
- *Visually perceived words are given expression in writing*: Exner's area (posterior part of 2nd frontal convolution).

21. What are the basic elements of language?

Ans. *Phonemes*: Smallest units of sound recognizable as language.
Morphemes: Smallest meaningful units of a word.
Syntax: Sentence structure.

22. What is dysphasia?

Ans. Dysphasia is a loss or impairment of the production and/ or comprehension of spoken or written language due to an acquired lesion of the brain.

23. What is dysarthria?

Ans. Dysarthria is a defect in articulation with intact mental functions and comprehension of spoken and written language and normal syntax (grammatical construction of sentence).

24. What is dysphonia?

Ans. Dysphonia is an alteration or loss of voice due to a disorder of the larynx or its innervations.

25. What is the normal number of words spoken per minute?

Ans. The normal number of words spoken per minute is 100 to 115 words per minute.

26. What is Broca's aphasia?

Ans. Speech in Broca's aphasia is sparse (10 to 15 words per minute).

27. What is neologism?

Ans. Syllables or words that are not part of the language.

28. What is jargon aphasia?

Ans. Fluent, paraphasic speech may be entirely incomprehensible.

29. What is global or total aphasia?

Ans. All aspects of speech and language being affected is called as global or total aphasia.

30. What are disconnection syndromes?

Ans. This term refers to certain disorders of language that result not from the lesions of the cortical areas themselves but from an apparent interruption of association pathways joining the primary receptive (sensory) areas to the language areas.

Conduction aphasias: Aphasias due to lesions that separate the more strictly receptive parts of the language itself from the purely motor ones.

Transcortical aphasias: Lesions that isolate the perisylvian language areas separating them from the other parts of the cerebral cortex.

- The identifying feature of these language disorders is a preservation of the ability to repeat.
- Preservation of the direct connection (arcuate fasciculus) is said to account for the ability to repeat.
- **Echolalia:** Tendency to repeat may be excessive.

31. What is conduction aphasia?

Ans.   i. Clinically severely impaired repetition.
  ii. Usual cause of conduction aphasia is an embolic occlusion of the ascending parietal or posterior temporal branch of MCA.
  iii. Lesions:
    a. Arcuate fasciculus
    b. Supramarginal gyrus
    c. Insula.

32. What is alexia without agraphia?

Ans.   i. The most striking feature of this syndrome is the retained capacity to write fluently after which the patient cannot read what has been written.
  ii. In most lesions confined to the posterior portion of the corpus callosum (splenium), only the visual part of the disconnection syndrome occurs. Occlusion of the left posterior cerebral artery is the example. Because infarction of the left occipital lobe causes a right homonymous

hemianopia, all visual information needed for activating the speech areas of the left hemisphere must therefore come from the right occipital lobe. The patient with a lesion of the spelenium of the corpus callosum or the adjacent white matter cannot read or name colours because the visual information cannot reach the left language areas. There is however, no difficulty in copying words; presumably the visual information for activating left motor area crosses the corpus callosum more anteriorly. Spontaneous writing and writing to dictation are also intact because the language areas are intact and interconnected, but after a delay, the patient is unable to read what he has previously written.

33. What is alexia with agraphia?

Ans. *Syndrome of the angular gyrus*: The lesion is confined to the angular gyrus and alexia may be combined with agraphia and other elements of the Werstmann syndrome.

34. What is pure-word deafness?

Ans.
   i. It is characterized by an impairment of auditory comprehension and repetition and an inability to write to dictation.

   ii. Non-verbal sounds such as doorbell can be heard without difficulty.

   iii. Ability to comprehend written language and spontaneous writing are preserved.

   iv. **Lesion:** Bilateral or left middle of the superior temporal gyrus.

35. What is foreign accent syndrome?

Ans. It is encountered as a transient phenomenon during recovery from stroke.

36. What is Pitre's law?

Ans. The language most used before the onset of aphasia will recover first. This is known as Pitre's law.

37. How is the brain function organized in the longitudinal oriented manner?

Ans. Brain functions are organized in three longitudinal oriented zones.

- A central vegetative neuronal system (allocortex and hypothalamus) provides the mechanisms for all internal functions (Milieu interior).

- An outer zone comprising the sensorimotor and association cortices providing the mechanisms for perceiving the external world.

- A region between them (limbic – paralimbic cortices) provides the bridges that permit the adaptation of organizational needs to the external environment.

38. What is neocortex?

Ans. Neocortex is recent cortex. It has uniform embryogenesis and morphology.

39. What is allocortex?

Ans. Allocortex is older cortex. It includes hippocampus and olfactory cortex.

40. What is homotypical cortex and heterotypical cortex?

Ans. *Homotypical cortex*: Six-layered arrangement is readily discerned.

Heterotypical cortex: Layers are less distinct, e.g. association cortex.

41. What is granular cortex?

Ans. i. Marked predominance of granular cells.

ii. Strongly developed for the receipt of afferent impulses.

iii. Seen in post-central gyrus, visual cortex and auditory areas.

42. What is agranular cortex?

Ans. When the precentral cortex is dominated by pyramidal rather than granular cells, this is called arganular cortex.

43. What are cortical tropisms or automatisms?

Ans. i. Automatisms or cortical tropisms are normally inhibited by frontal cortex.

ii. Destruction of particular areas disinhibits or releases other areas, e.g. destruction of pre-motor areas leaving precentral and parietal lobes intact result in release of sensorimotor automatisms such as groping, grasping and sucking.

44. Discuss the clinical anatomy of frontal lobe.

Ans. *Area 4*: Primary motor cortex

Area 6: Supplementary motor cortex

Area 8: Turning the eyes and head contralaterally

Area 44: Broca's speech area

Cingulate gyrus: Limbic system

Prefrontal cortex: 9 to 12, 45 to 47

a. Initiation of planned action

b. Executive control of all mental operations including emotional expressions.

45. What are the clinical effects of frontal lobe lesions?

Ans. 1. Motor abnormalities related to the prerolandic motor cortex.

2. Speech and language disorders related to the dominant hemisphere.

3. Incontinence of bladder and bowel.

4. Impairment of certain cognitive functions especially attention, concentration, capacity for sustained mental activity and ability to shift from one line of thought or action to another, i.e. both impersistence and perservation.

5. Akinesia and lack of initiative and spontaneity (apathy and abulia).

6. Other changes in personality particularly in mood and self-control (disinhibition of behaviour).

7. A distinctive abnormality of gait.

46. What is the blood supply to the frontal lobe?

Ans. 1. Blood is supplied to the medial parts of the frontal lobe by the anterior cerebral artery.

2. Blood is supplied to the convexity and deep regions by the superior (rolandic) division of the middle cerebral artery.

47. What is the clinical anatomy of temporal lobes?

Ans. 1. *Transversi gyri of Heschl*: Located within the sylvian fissure, primary auditory receptive area.

2. *Planum temporale (area 22)*: Left planum is larger in right handed individuals.

3. *Areas 21 and 37*: For learning and vision.

4. *Superior part of the non-dominant temporal lobe*: Spatial orientation.

5. *Hippocampal formation*: Concerned with (a) learning, (b) memory, (c) olfactory system, (d) unlike the six-layered neocortex, the hippocampus and dentate gyrus are typical of the phylogenetically older three layered allocortex.

48. What are the clinical effects of temporal lobe lesions?

Ans. 1. *Visual disorders*

  a. Kluver-Bucy syndrome:
   • Compulsions to attend to all visual stimuli
   • Hyperorality
   • Hypersexuality
   • Blunted emotional reactivity

  b. Complex visual hallucinations

2. *Auditory disorders*

  a. Cortical deafness (similar to Anton's syndrome)

  b. Auditory agnosias
   • Non-dominant hemisphere is important for harmony and melody aspects of music.
   • Dominant hemisphere is important for writing and reading aspects of music.

c. Word-deafness (auditory verbal agnosia): Wernicke's aphasia

d. Auditory hallucinations and illusions
  - Dominant temporal lobe: Impairment in tests of verbal material presented through the auditory sense.
  - Non-dominant temporal lobe: Impairment in tests of visually presented non-verbal material.

3. *Vestibular disturbances*
4. *Time perception*
5. *Smell, taste, memory, emotion, behaviour.*

49. What is the blood supply to the temporal lobes?

Ans. i. The inferior branch of the middle cerebral artery supplies the convexity of the temporal lobe.

ii. Temporal branch of the posterior cerebral artery supplies the medial and inferior aspects including the hippo-campus.

50. What is the blood supply to the parietal lobe?

Ans. The parietal lobe is supplied by the middle cerebral artery, the inferior and superior divisions supplying the inferior and superior lobules respectively.

51. What is agnosia?

Ans. Agnosia refers to a loss of recognition of an entity that cannot be attributed to a defect in the primary sensory modality.

52. What are the clinical effects of parietal lobe lesions?

Ans. 1. *Cortical sensory syndromes*
  - Sensory discrimination (tactile localization, 2-point discrimination, barognosis, stereognosis, graphesthesia).
  - Bilaterally sensory disturbance in nearly half of the patients with unilateral lesions, but the deficits are more severe contralaterally and mainly in the hand.
  - Tactile inattention or extinction: Disregard of stimuli on the affected side when the healthy side is stimulated simultaneously.

2. *Asomatognosia*: Asomatognosia denotes the inability to recognize part of one's body. Visual and tactile sensory information is synthesized during development into a body scheme or image (perception of one's body and the relations of bodily parts to one another).

3. *Anosognosia*
   - The patient with a dense hemiplegia usually of the left side may be indifferent to the paralysis or unaware of it.
   - Unilateral asomatognosia is seven times as frequent with right (non-dominant) parietal lesions as with left sided ones.
   - Allocheria: One sided stimulus is felt on the other side.
   - Sensory extinction, dressing apraxia, constructional apraxia.
   - Amorphosynthesis: An inability to summate a series of spatial impressions—tactile, kinesthetic, visual or auditory.
   - Gerstmann syndrome: Bilateral asomatognosia
   Lesion: Inferior parietal lobule (angular gyrus) dominant hemisphere.
   a. Finger agnosia
   b. Confusion of sides
   c. Dyscalculia
   d. Dysgraphia
   - Superior parietal lobule lesion: Optic ataxia

4. *Ideomotor and ideational apraxia*: Patients with parietal lesions of the dominant hemisphere who exhibit no deficits in motor or sensory functions lose the ability to perform learned motor skills on command or by imitation.

5. *Visual disorders with parietal lesions*
   - Optokinetic nystagmus is abolished
   - Left sided visual neglect
   - *Topographagnosia*: Patients with this disorder are unable to orient themselves in an abstract spatial setting.
   - *Lesion*: Dorsal convexity of the right parietal lobe.

6. *Auditory neglect*
   Lesion: Right superior lobule.

53. What is the blood supply to the occipital lobe? Explain macular sparing?

Ans. i. A majority of occipital lobe gets blood supply by posterior cerebral artery.

ii. A small area of the occipital pole receives blood supply from the inferior division of the middle cerebral artery. This explains macular sparing.

54. What are the clinical effects of occipital lobe lesions?

Ans. 1. Visual field defects

- Macular splitting: A lesion confined to the pole of the occipital lobe results in central hemianopic defect that splits the macular area and leaves the peripheral fields intact
- Cortical blindness, asthenopia (visual fatigue)
- Anton's syndrome: Visual anosognosia
- Visual illusions (metamorphopsias)
  - Polyopia (one object appearing as two or more objects)
  - Palinopsia (perseveration of visual image)
- *Visual hallucinations*:
  - Elementary or unformed hallucinations: Calcarine cortex
  - Complex (formed) hallucinations: Visual association areas or their connections with the temporal lobe.

2. Visual agnosias

- Visual object agnosia: Cannot even tell the generic class of the object presented. Visual object recognition consists of two distinct processes
  - a. *Apperception*: Construction of a perceptual representation from vision.
  - b. Mapping of this perceptual representation onto stored percepts or engrams of the objects functions and associations.
    - *Simultanagnosia*: Patient recognizes parts but not the whole.
    - *Balint's syndrome*: Faults in ocular scanning might underlie all the defects.

Components:

a. Simultanagnosia

b. *Optic ataxia*: Difficulty in touching an object under visual guidance as though hand and eye are not co-ordinated.

c. *Optic apraxia*: An inability to project gaze voluntarily into the peripheral field and to scan it despite the fact that eye movements are full.

d. *Lesion*: Bilateral often between areas 19 and 7.

- *Prosopagnosia*: Inability to identify faces.
- *Lesion*: Bilateral lesions of the ventromesial occipito-temporal regions.
- *Environmental agnosia*: Gets lost when faced with the actual landscape.
- *Lesion*: Right sided medial temporo-occipital region.
- Visual agnosia for words (alexia without agraphia).
- *Colour agnosia*:

Central achromatopsia: Acquired colour blindness due to a cerebral lesion with retention of colour vision.

55. What are the disturbances of the non-dominant cerebral hemisphere?

Ans. It is in the sphere of visuospatial perception that right hemi-spheral dominance is most convincing.

a. Constructional apraxia

b. Topographic agnosia

c. Prosopagnosia

d. Simultanagnosia.

56. Name the various disconnection syndromes.

Ans. They are:

- Inter-hemispheric disconnection
- Intra-hemispheric disconnection.

57. Discuss inter-hemispheric disconnection (alexia without agraphia).

Ans. *Alexia*: Lesion—infarction of the left occipital lobe.

Since the infarction of the left occipital lobe causes a right homonymous hemianopia, all visual information needed for activating the speech areas of the left hemisphere must therefore come from the right occipital lobe. The patient with a lesion of the splenium of the corpus callosum or the adjacent white matter cannot read or name colour because the visual information cannot reach the left language areas.

Without agraphia: There is however no difficulty in copying words presumably the visual information for activating the left motor area crosses the corpus callosum more anteriorly.

58. What are intra-hemispheric disconnections?

Ans. 1. *Conduction aphasia*: Impaired repetition but good comprehension and fluency because Wernicke's area is separated from Broca's area by a lesion in arcuate fasciculus or supramarginal gyrus.

2. *Ideomotor (sympathetic) apraxia in Broca's aphasia*
   Lesion: Left frontal lobe underlying white matter causing left limb apraxia, i.e. apraxia of the non-paralyzed hand.
   If the lesion in the deep white matter separates the language area from the right motor cortex but not from the left, the patient can write correctly with the right hand and aphasically with the left.

3. *Pure word deafness*
   Lesion: Subcortical lesion of the left temporal lobe sparing Wernicke's area and interrupting also those auditory fibres that cross in the corpus callous from the opposite side. Thus, there is a failure to articulate the left auditory language area (Wernicke's area).
   Although the patient is able to hear and identify non-verbal sounds, there is a loss of ability to discriminate speech sounds, i.e. to comprehend spoken language.

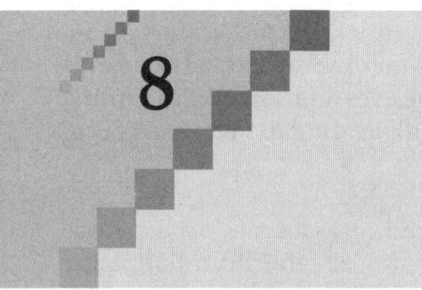

8

Epilepsy

1. What is epilepsy?

Ans. Epilepsy is described as a condition in which a person has recurrent seizures due to chronic underlying process. Epilepsy has two or more unprovoked seizures.

2. What is convulsion?

Ans. It is intense paroxysms of involuntary repetitive muscular contractions.

3. What is seizure?

Ans. It is a paroxysmal event due to abnormal, excessive hyper synchronous discharge from an aggregate of CNS neurons.

4. What are partial seizures?

Ans. i. A partial seizure means that the electrical abnormality is localized to one part of the brain.

ii. Usually associated with a structural abnormality in the brain.

iii. Jacksonian march, Todd's paralysis, complex partialis continua are additional features.

iv. It may then spread and become a generalized seizure.

5. What is Jacksonian epilepsy?

Ans. Some attacks begin in one part (e.g. mouth, thumb, great toe, etc.) and spread gradually to other parts. This is known as Jacksonian epilepsy.

6. What is versive seizure?

Ans. A frontal epileptic focus may involve the frontal eye fields causing forced deviation of the eyes and sometimes turning of the head to the opposite side leading to versive seizure.

7. What is Todd's paralysis?

Ans. Epileptic attacks with prolonged episodes may leave paresis of the involved limb lasting for several hours after the seizure ceases (an overshoot of inhibitory mechanisms). This is known as Todd's paralysis.

8. What is kindling?

Ans. Cells undergoing repetitive epileptic discharges undergo morphological and physiological changes which make them likely to produce subsequent abnormal discharges.

9. What are complex partial seizures?

Ans. It is a partial seizure with loss of awareness. The behavioral arrest is usually accompanied by automatisms which are involuntary automatic behaviors that has a wide range of manifestations.

10. Describe absence seizure.

Ans. i. If the abnormal electrical activity fails to affect muscle tone.
ii. Consciousness is lost but the patient remains standing or sitting.
iii. Absence attacks are caused by a generalized discharge that does not spread off the hemisphere and so does not cause loss of posture.
iv. It is not associated with postictal confusion.
v. It usually begins in childhood (age 4 to 8 yr) or early adolescence and are the main seizure types in 15 to 20% of children with epilepsy.
vi. The electrophysiological hallmark of typical absence seizure is a generalized symmetric 3 HZ spike and wave discharge that begins and ends suddenly, superimposed on a normal EEG background.

vii. 60 to 70% of such patients will have a spontaneous remission during adolescence.

11. In which type of epilepsy is CT head not required?

Ans. CT head is not required in absence epilepsy.

12. What is a mirror focus?

Ans. A seizure focus if active for a time, may sometimes establish via a commissural connection, a persistent secondary focus in the corresponding cortical areas of the opposite hemisphere. This is known as mirror focus.

13. Describe febrile seizures.

Ans.
i. Febrile seizures are seizures associated with fever but without evidence of CNS infection or other defined causes.
ii. Febrile seizures occur between 3 months and 5 years of age and has a peak incidence between 18 and 24 months.
iii. Prevalence is 3 to 5%.
iv. The seizures are likely to occur during the rising phase of the temperature curve (i.e. during the first day) rather than well into the course of the illness.
v. A simple febrile seizure is a single, isolated event, brief and symmetric in appearance.
   Complex febrile seizures are characterized by:
   a. Repeated activity
   b. Duration more than 15 minutes
   c. Focal features.
   Treatment of febrile seizures: Diazepam
   Prophylaxis: Phenobarbitone for 2 to 3 years.

14. What is catamenial epilepsy?

Ans. Epilepsy occurring during menstrual periods in women is called catamenial epilepsy.
Acetazolamide (250 to 500 mg/day) may be effective as adjuvant therapy in some cases when started 7 to 10 days prior to the onset of menses and continued until bleeding stops.

15. What are myoclonic seizures?

Ans. Myoclonus is a sudden and brief muscular contraction that may involve one part of the body or the entire body. It occurs in two ways:

Physiological: Sudden jerking movement while falling asleep.

Pathological:

a. Metabolic disorders

b. Degenerative CNS disease

c. Anoxic brain injury.

16. What are atonic and purely tonic seizures?

Ans. They only occur in the context of epilepsy syndrome with other forms of seizures. They are associated with epileptic syndrome, e.g. tonic type in Lennox–Gastaut syndrome.

17. What is the age group when epileptic seizures begin?

Ans. Over two-thirds of all epileptic seizures begin in childhood (mostly in the first year of life). This is the age period when seizures assume the widest array of forms.

18. What biochemical abnormality confirms organic seizures?

Ans. i. Serum prolactin

ii. Serum prolactin level rises after 10 to 20 minutes after all types of seizures except:

• Absence seizure

• Myoclonic type.

19. How is Ictal SPECT useful?

Ans. It shows hyperperfusion of the seizure focus.

20. What is the most common histological finding in brain of epileptics?

Ans. Bilateral loss of neurons in the CA segment of hippocampus.

21. What is SUDEP?

Ans. i. Sudden unexpected death in epileptic patients.

ii. It usually affects young people with convulsive seizures and tends to occur at night.

iii. SUDEP may result from brain stem-mediated effects of seizures on cardiac rhythms or pulmonary functions.

22. What is epileptic syndrome?

Ans. Epileptic syndromes are disorders in which epilepsy is a predominant feature and there is sufficient evidence, (e.g. through clinical, EEG, radiological or genetic observation) to suggest a common underlying mechanism.

23. What are the causes and manifestations of symptomatic generalized epilepsies?

Ans. *Causes*:
- Prematurity
- Prenatal injury
- Metabolic disorders of infancy

Manifestations: West syndrome progress to Lennox-Gastaut syndrome.

West syndrome:
- Infantile spasms
- Characteristic EEG abnormality (3 Hz hypsarrhythmias)
- Arrest in mental development.

Lennox-Gastaut syndrome:
- Combination of seizures
- Distinct slow (1-2 HZ) spike and wave EEG pattern
- Progressive intellectual impairment.

24. What are the special epileptic syndromes?

Ans. i. Benign childhood epilepsy with centrotemporal spike and epilepsy with occipital spike

ii. Infantile spasms: Clonazepam is probably the most widely used

iii. Febrile seizures, reflex epilepsy

iv. Epilepsy partialis continua

v. Hysterical seizure.

25. What is the treatment of neonatal seizures?

Ans. i. Pyridoxine (vitamin B_6) deficiency is an important cause of neonatal seizures.

Treatment: Intramuscular pyridoxine 25–50 mg.

ii. Phenytoin should not be used because of immaturity of the hepatic hydroxylating system responsible for phenytoin detoxification.

Treatment: Phenobarbitone is preferred (15–20 mg/kg).

iii. *Lennox-Gastaut syndrome*: Valproic acid (900 to 2400 mg) will reduce the frequency of spells in approximately half the cases.

iv. *Infantile spasms*
Treatment:
- ACTH
- Adrenal corticosteroids
- Vigabartin.

26. Discuss single seizure.

Ans. i. One-third of patients with a single unprovoked seizure will have another seizure within 5 years.

ii. The risk of seizure is greater if:
- Seizure is present in sibling.
- Complex partial seizure is present in childhood.
- Spike and wave abnormality in EEG.

Treatment: Administer anti-convulsants for 6–12 months and then re-evaluate.

27. What is the correlation of stroke with seizure?

Ans. Acute seizures (i.e. occurring at the time when strokes are seen most often with embolic rather than haemorrhage or thrombotic strokes.

28. What are the risk factors for recurrent seizure?

Ans. i. An abnormal neurological examination

ii. Seizure presenting as status epilepticus

iii. Postictal Todd's paralysis

iv. Strong family history of seizures

v. An abnormal EEG.

29. What are the differentiating points between seizure and syncope?

Ans. i. Postictal confusion

ii. Incontinence

iii. Tongue biting

iv. Elevated prolactin level.

30. What is paroxysmal depolarization shift?

Ans. Intracelluar recordings show bursts of rapid action potential firing with reduction of trans-membrane potential.

31. What is the EEG pattern in GTCS?

Ans. i. *Tonic phase*: High amplitude spike.

ii. *Clonic activity*: Slow wave to create spike and wave pattern.

32. What are the EEG changes during seizure initiation?

Ans. i. High frequency bursts of action potential.

ii. Hyper-synchronization.

33. How frequent are interictal changes in EEG?

Ans. i. Interictal changes of EEG in epilepsy is 30–50%.

ii. With activation procedure, it is 60–70%.

34. What are the general guidelines for treatment of epilepsy?

Ans. i. Higher serum concentration of drugs are necessary for the control of simple or complex partial seizures than for the control of tonic clonic seizures alone.

ii. Sodium valproate and carbamazepine should not be used because the inhibition of epoxide hydrolase by valproic acid leads to toxicity through the build up of carbamazepine epoxide.

iii. Saturation kinetics of phenytoin: Phenytoin shows saturation kinetics such that small increase in phenytoin doses above a standard maintenance dose can precipitate marked side-effect. Example: A typical increase in dose from 300 to 400 mg daily often results in a disproportionate elevation of the serum levels and toxic side-effects.

    iv. Carbamazepine induces its own metabolism and therefore doses adequate to control seizures at the outset of therapy are no longer effective several weeks later.

    v. Treatment of juvenile myoclonic epilepsy is lifelong.

    vi. Carbamazepine and valproate are probably preferable to phenytion for epileptic children because they do not cause facial features and do not produce gum hypertrophy or breast enlargement.

    vii. Because of the high incidence of myoclonic epilepsy in adolescence, it is the practice to use valproate as the first drug in this age group.

    viii. Commonly used anti-epileptic drugs increase risk of fracture from osteoporosis due to degradation of vitamin D and hence calcium supplements are advised.

35. When is polypharmacy useful?

Ans. i. Approximately one-third of patients with epilepsy do not respond to treatment with a single AED and it becomes necessary to try a combination of drugs to control seizures.

    ii. Patients likely to require multiple drugs are:

      a. Focal epilepsy related to an underlying structural lesion

      b. Multiple seizure types

      c. Developmental delay.

36. Discuss newer anti-epileptic drugs.

Ans. i. *Lamotrigine*

      a. Prevents the release of glutamate

      b. Causes skin rash

      c. Alternative to valproate in young women

      d. It appears to be effective in epilepsy syndromes with mixed generalized seizure types such as JME and Lennox-Gastaut syndrome

    ii. *Levitiracetam*

      a. Novel sodium channel blocker

      b. Treatment of partial seizures

      c. Produces sleepiness and dizziness

iii. *Felbamate*
    a. It causes bone marrow suppressio
    b. It causes liver failure
iv. *Gabapentin and pregabalin*: It enhances GABA.
 v. *Topiramate*: It causes renal stones.

37. What are the common side-effects of anti-epileptic drugs?

Ans. Almost all commonly used AEDs cause dose related side-effects.
    i. Sedation
    ii. Ataxia
    iii. Diplopia.

38. What is the risk of subsequent seizure after a single seizure?

Ans. 40%.

39. What is the recurrence rate of seizure after drug withdrawal?

Ans. 40%

40. What are the anti-epileptic drugs which cause renal stones?

Ans. i. Acetazolamide
    ii. Topiramate
    iii. Zonisamide

41. What is the AED which is associated with hyponatremia?

Ans. Carbamazepine.

42. What is the correlation of AED with oral contraception?

Ans. Phenytoin and carbamazepine are not ideal agents for a young woman wishing to use oral contraception because the drugs induce liver enzymes and therefore oral contraceptives may become ineffective.

43. Discuss AED and teratogenic effects.

Ans. • *Midface hypoplasia*: Shortened nose, pheltrum, inner canthal distance and finger hypoplasia are characteristics of AED exposure.

Teratogenic effects:
- In pregnancy, the preferred AED is phenytoin.
- Neural tube defects are greatest with valproate.

44. Which AED does not cause teratogenicity?
Ans. Gabapentin does not cause teratogenicity.

45. How to treat coagulopathy in the fetus exposed to pheno-barbitone?
Ans. *Mother*: Oral vitamin K 20 mg/day during eight months or 10 mg. IV four hours before birth
Neonate: 1 mg im to the neonate.

46. What is eclampsia? How is it treated?
Ans. Eclampsia is a form of hypertensive encephalopathy (hypertension plus convulsion)
Treatment: Magnesium sulphate 4 gm IV over 5 to 10 minutes followed by a maintenance dose of 5 gm every four hours IM.

47. Should AEDs be continued during pregnancy?
Ans. Since the potential harm of uncontrolled seizures on the mother and fetus is considered greater than the teratogenic effects of AEDs, it is currently recommended that pregnant women be maintained on effective drug therapy.

48. Discuss sodium valproate.
Ans. i. It causes weight gain and menstrual irregularities.
   ii. It causes neural tube defects in fetuses of pregnant woman.
   iii. Hepatotoxic in children below 2 years of age.
   iv. *It can be given as IV preparation*: Maximum recommended rate of administration is 20 mg/minute.
   v. The dose of sodium valproate in status epilepticus is 10 mg/kg IV over 3 to 5 minutes and 800 to 1000 mg/day.

49. Discuss status epilepticus.
Ans. i. It is recurrent generalized convulsions at a frequency that prevents regaining of consciousness in the interval between seizures.

ii. Overall mortality is 25%

iii. It is an emergency because it can cause

  a. Cardiorespiratory dysfunction

  b. Hyperthermia

  c. Metabolic derangements

iv. Treatment:

  a. *Immediate suppression of convulsions*: Lorazepam or diazepam 2 to 4 mg/min IV to a total dose of 10 to 15 mg.

  b. *Loading with anti-convulsants*: Phenytoin 15-20 mg/kg IV at 25–50 mg/min in normal saline or fosphenytoin at 50 to 75 mg/min.

50. What are the most common causes of status epilepticus?

Ans. i. Anti-convulsant withdrawal or non-compliance

ii. Metabolic derangement

iii. Drug toxicity

iv. CNS infections

v. CNS tumours

vi. Refractory epilepsy

vii. Head trauma.

51. What is acute repetitive seizure?

Ans. The patient's awakeness between fits is known as acute repetitive seizure.

Treatment:

i. Diazepam rectal gel

ii. Nasal or buccal midazolam.

52. How to treat petitmal status?

Ans. i. IV lorazepam

ii. Valproic acid or both followed by ethosuximide.

53. What is the treatment of non-convulsive status?

Ans. Treatment is along the lines of grandmal status usually stopping short of anesthetic agents.

54. What is ketogenic diet?

Ans. i. Starvation for a day or two in order to induce ketones followed by a diet in which 80 to 90% of the calories are derived from fat.

ii. The diet can be effective in refractory cases of epilepsy in childhood.

55. What is vagus nerve stimulation?

Ans. i. Stimulation of vagus nuclei leads to widespread activation of cortical and subcortical pathways and are associated with increased seizure threshold.

ii. Used in intractable partial or secondary generalized seizure.

iii. Stimulating electrodes are connected to the vagus at the left carotid bifurcation.

56. What percent of epilepsy need surgery?

Ans. Approximately 20% of patients with epilepsy are resistant to medical therapy and therefore may need surgery.

9

Involuntary Movements and Gait

1. Discuss physio-anatomic considerations of basal ganglia.

Ans. There are two pathways:

1. *Direct pathway*
   a. It facilitates movement.
   b. Decreased conduction through direct pathway decreases movement, e.g. Parkinson's disease.
2. *Indirect pathway*
   a. It impedes voluntary movement.
   b. Decreased conduction through indirect pathway facilitates movement, e.g. Huntington's disease.

2. What are dopamine receptors?

Ans. There are two families:

D_1 *family (D_1 and D_5 subtypes)*: Acts through direct neurons.
D_2 *family (D_{2-4} subtypes)*: Acts through indirect neurons.

3. What is gegenhalten?

Ans. Connections of the basal ganglia to the frontal lobe are impaired causing a distinctive type of variable resistance in which the patient seems unable to relax a group of muscles on request.

4. What is chorea?

Ans. Chorea (dance) refers to involuntary arrhythmic movements of a forcible rapid jerky type.

Examples:
  i. Huntington
  ii. Sydenhams
  iii. Neuroleptics (phenothiazines).

5. What is athetosis (unfixed/changeable)?

Ans. The maintained posture is interrupted by relatively slow, sinuous, purposeless movements that have a tendency to flow into one another. The abnormal movements are most pronounced in digits, hands, face, tongue and throat.

6. What is ballismus?

Ans. Ballismus is an uncontrollable, poorly patterned flinging movement of an entire limb.
  Treatment: Halloperidol/phenothiazines.

7. What is dystonia?

Ans. It is a persistent attitude on posture produced by co-contraction of agonist and antagonist muscles that place the limb in an unnatural position. It especially involves large axial muscles (trunk and limb girdle).

8. What are the acute generalized dystonic reactions?

Ans. These reactions are caused by phenothiazines, butyro-phenones, metoclopramide, olanzipine. They are of two types.
  1. *Acute dystonic reactions*
    Treatment:
    a. Diphenhydramine
    b. Benzotropine (two or three times in 24 to 48 hours).
  2. *Tardive dyskinesias* (due to chronic usage) because of:
    a. Long standing use
    b. Withdrawal of medication.

9. What is the treatment of dystonias?

Ans. i. Trihexyphenidyl
  ii. Botulinum toxins: Focal dystonia.

10. Describe cerebellar functions in transverse and longitudinal manner.

Ans. 1. **Transverse (from posterior to anterior)**
   - *Spinocerebellum*: Posture and muscle tone, dysarthria.
   - *Pontocerebellum*: Co-ordination of skilled movements.
   - *Vestibulocerebellum*: Equilibrium and ocular movements.

   2. **Longitudinal (from central to lateral)**
   - *Vermian*: Co-ordinates the movements of the eyes and body (Gait).
   - *Paravermian*: Postural tone and dysarthria.
   - *Lateral*: Co-ordination of movements of ipsilateral limbs.

11. Why are cerebellar manifestations ipsilateral?

Ans. Since the pathway from the cerebellar nuclei to the thalamus and then onto the motor cortex is crossed and the connection from the motor cortex through the corticospinal tract is again crossed, the effects of lesions of one cerebellar hemisphere are manifested by the signs on the ipsilateral side of the body.

12. Why cerebellar nystagmus is a gaze evoked nystagmus?

Ans. i. The brain stem and cerebellum are involved in maintaining eccentric position of gaze.

   ii. Lesions will therefore allow eyes to drift back towards the primary position.

   iii. This produces nystagmus whose fast component beats in the direction of the gaze.

13. What is the etiology of cerebellar ataxia?

Ans. 1. *Acute transitory*: Alcohol, anti-convulsants

   2. *Acute and reversible*: Postinfectious, viral cerebellar encephalitis

   3. *Acute enduring*: Hyperthermia, post-anoxic, mercury compounds

4. *Subacute (over weeks)*
   a. Brain tumours
   b. Alcoholic
   c. Paraneoplastic
   d. Cerebellar abscess
5. *Chronic (months to years)*: Fredricke's ataxia and other spino-cerebellar degenerations.

14. What is tremor?

Ans. Tremor may be defined as a more or less involuntary and rhythmic oscillatory movement produced by alternating or irregular synchronous contractions of reciprocally innervated muscles.

- Its rhythmic quality distinguishes tremor from other involuntary movements.
- Involvement of agonist and antagonist muscles distinguish it from clonus.

15. What is the frequency of physiological and pathological tremor?

Ans. *Physiological tremor*: Frequency is 10 hertz.
Pathological tremor: Frequency is 5 hertz.

16. Describe essential tremor.

Ans. a. It is the commonest type of tremor.
     b. It is unassociated with other neurologic changes and is therefore essential.
     c. Frequency is 5 hertz.
     d. Maintenance of posture exaggerates these tremors.
     e. Alcohol ameliorates and anxiety exaggerates this tremor.

17. What is Negro's sign?

Ans. Cogwheel rigidity of Parkinson disease is known as Negro's sign.

18. Where is the lesion in palatal myoclonus?

Ans. Lesion is triangle of guillain and mollaret.

Treatment:
1. Clonazepam
2. Sodium valproate
3. Gabapentin.

19. What is asterixis?
Ans. Arrhythmic lapses of sustained posture is called asterixis.

20. What is clonus?
Ans. It refers to a series of rhythmic, monophasic (i.e. unidirectional) contractions and relaxations of a group of muscle, differing in this way from tremors which are always diphasic or bidirectional. ·

21. What is myoclonus?
Ans. It specifies the shock like contractions of a group of muscles, irregular in rhythm and amplitude.

22. What is myoclonus multiplex or polymyoclonus?
Ans. It is widespread, lightening like, arrhythmic contractions.

23. What are the causes of myoclonus?
Ans. a. Myoclonic epilepsies, e.g. MERRF
   b. Myoclonic dementias, e.g. CJD, SSPE
   c. Essential and heredofamilial forms
   d. Myoclonus with cerebellar disease
      Examples:
      1. Opsoclonus myoclonus (para-neoplastic)
      2. Post-anoxic myoclonus.
   e. *Metabolic and toxic disorders*: Uremia, lithium, hepatic encephalopathy.
   f. *Focal and spinal forms of myoclonus*:
      • Herpes zoster myelitis
      • Traumatic spinal cord injury.

24. What is the mechanism of myoclonus?
Ans. A lack of modulatory influence of the cerebellum on the thalamocortical system of neurons has been postulated as a likely mechanism.

25. What is the characteristic feature of Tay-Sach's disease?

Ans. Each auditory stimulus results in blinking, abrupt elevation of the arms and other movements. This audiogenic form of sensory myoclonus is characteristic of Tay-Sach's disease.

26. What is the treatment of blepharospasm?

Ans. 1. L-Dopa
2. Botulinum toxin
3. Anti-cholinergic drugs.

27. What is tardive dyskinesia?

Ans. Abnormal movements are due to the hypersensitivity of dopamine receptors in the basal ganglia, secondary to prolonged blockade of the receptors by anti-pyschotic medications. It refers specifically to movements induced by the anti-pyschotic drugs usually phenothiazine that persist after the drugs are withdrawn.
Treatment is with newer atypical anti-psychotic drugs (clozapine, quitapine).

28. What are tics and habit spasms?

Ans. 1. Stereotypy and
2. Irresistibility are the main identifying features of these phenomena.

29. Describe Gilles de la Tourette syndrome. Why is this syndrome uncommon in Japanese patients?

Ans. 1. Distinguishing features are:
   a. Multiplicity of tics
   b. Combination of motor and vocal tics
2. Coprolalia: Compulsive utterance of obscenities are the most dramatic manifestations. Interestingly they are uncommon in Japanese patients whose decorous culture and language contain few obscenities.
3. L-Dopa exacerbates the symptoms of tourette syndrome and haloperidol which blocks dopamine (particularly D_2) receptors, is an effective treatment.

30. What is akathesia?

Ans. An inner feeling of restlessness, an inability to sit still and a compulsion to move about caused by neuroleptic drugs, L-dopa, psychiatric disorders.

31. Which drug is commonly implicated in vestibular dysfunction?

Ans. Aminoglycoside antibiotics are commonly implicated in vestibular dysfunction.

32. What is Rhomberg's sign?

Ans. i. It is due to abnormalities in proprioceptive sensibilities.
ii. When standing if instructed to close the eyes, they sway markedly and fall.

33. What happens when there is vermian (midline) cerebellar lesion?

Ans. a. Control of gait is impaired.
b. Signs of cerebellar inco-ordination of arms and legs are NOT impaired.

34. What happens when there are bilateral cerebellar lesions?

Ans. There is often titubation (tremor) of the head and trunk.

35. What are the causes of sensory ataxia (lesion of the posterior column) which causes stamping of the feet?

Ans. a. Tabetic foot (tabes dorsalis)
b. Friedrich's ataxia and spinocerebellar degeneration
c. Subacute combined degeneration of the cord
d. Syphilitic meningomyelitis
e. Chronic sensory polyneuropathies
f. Multiple sclerosis
g. Compression of the spinal cord (spondylosis and meningioma) in which the posterior columns are predominantly involved.

36. What is high-stepping gait?

Ans. 1. This is caused by paralysis of the pretibial and peroneal muscle with resultant inability to dorsiflex and evert the foot (foot drop).

2. Foot drop occurs in diseases that affect the peripheral nerves of the leg or motor neurons in the spinal cord such as
   • Chronic acquired neuropathies (diabetes, inflammatory, toxic, nutritional)
   • Charcot marie tooth disease (peroneal muscular atrophy)
   • Progressive spinal muscular atrophy
   • Poliomyelitis
3. Certain types of muscular dystrophy in which the distal musculature of the limb is involved.

37. What is cerebellar gait? Where is it seen?

Ans. Cerebellar gait is an ataxic gait. It is most commonly seen in patients with
   • Multiple sclerosis
   • Cerebellar tumours (particularly those affecting the vermis disproportionately, e.g. medulloblastoma)
   • Stroke (ischaemic and haemorrhagic)
   • **Most dramatically:** Cerebellar degenerations.

38. What are hemiplegic and paraplegic gaits?

Ans. Hemiplegic gait causes circumduction.
   Paraplegic gait causes scissors gait:
   A bilateral hemiplegic gait affects only the lower limbs.

39. What is festinating gait?

Ans. i. Festinating gait is seen in Parkinson's disease patients.
   ii. Festinate is a Latin word meaning to hasten.

40. What is the gait disorder in normal pressure hydrocephalus?

Ans. These patients are able to carry-out the movements of stepping while supine or sitting but have difficulty in taking steps when upright or attempting to walk.

41. What is astasia-abasia?

Ans. i. It is hysterical gait.
   ii. Patients though unable to either stand or walk display more or less normal use of their legs while in bed and have an otherwise normal neurological examination.

10

Dementia, Sleep and Related Disorders

1. What is dementia?

Ans. Dementia is defined as a deterioration of cognitive abilities and intelligence with little or no disturbances of consciousness or perception.

It is an acquired deterioration in cognitive abilities that impair the successful performance of activities of daily living.

2. What is amnesia?

Ans. It is a term used to describe an impairment in memory function.

3. What is executive function?

Ans. i. It refers to mental activity involved in planning, initiating and regulating behavior (systematic and goal directed activity).

ii. Executive functions are presumed to involve the frontal lobe.

4. What is Capgra's syndrome?

Ans. It is a delusion that a familiar person has been replaced by an imposter. Approximately 10% of Alzheimer disease patients develop Capgra's syndrome.

5. What is intelligence?

Ans. To act purposefully, to think rationally and to deal effectively with his environment is intelligence.

6. What is Ribot's law of memory?

Ans. Up to a certain period in the illness, memories of the distant past are relatively well retained at a time when more recently acquired information has been lost. This is known as Ribot's law of memory.

7. What are cortical and subcortical dementias?

Ans. a. *Cortical dementia (e.g. Alzheimer's disease)*
- Prominent disturbances of memory, language and calculation
- Prominent signs of apraxia and agnosia
- Impaired capacity for abstract thought.

b. *Subcortical dementia (e.g. basal ganglia disease)*
- Motility disorders and involuntary movements
- Language (vocabulary, naming) and praxis are spared
- Degrees of forgetfulness, slowed thought process, lack of initiative and depression of mood.

8. What is bedside classification of dementias?

Ans. 1. Disease in which dementia is associated with clinical and laboratory signs of other medical diseases, e.g. hypothyroidism.

2. Diseases in which dementia is associated with neurologic signs but not with other obvious medical diseases, e.g. Huntington's chorea.

3. Disease in which dementia is usually the only evidence of neurologic or medical disease, e.g. Alzheimer's disease.

9. What are the treatable forms of dementia?

Ans. a. Subdural haematoma
b. Certain brain tumors
c. Chronic drug intoxication
d. Normal pressure hydrocephalus
e. AIDS (reversible to some extent)
f. Neurosyphilis
g. Cryptococcosis

h. Pellagra
i. Vitamin B$_{12}$ deficiency
j. Thiamine deficiency
k. Hypothyroidism
l. Other metabolic and endocrine disorders.

10. What is the surest sign of metabolic or drug induced encephalopathy?

Ans. Asterexis.

11. Can seizures occur in degenerative dementia?

Ans. Usually not. Seizures are not a usual component of the degenerative dementias.

12. What is retrograde amnesia?

Ans. It is an impaired ability to recall events and other information that has been firmly established before the onset of illness.

13. What is anterograde amnesia?

Ans. It is an impaired ability to acquire certain types of new information, i.e. to learn or to form new memories.

14. What are procedural and declarative memory?

Ans. Procedural memory is knowing how.
Declarative memory is knowing what.

15. What are the neuropsychological categories of memory?

Ans. i. Immediate recall (repetition)
ii. Working memory (short-term recall of objects, place name, sequencing)
iii. Long-term memory
• *Explicit*:
a. *Semantic*: Recall for facts and their temporal relationships
b. *Episodic*: Recall for temporarily organized events
• *Implicit*:
a. *Procedural*: Operational recall (how to do)
b. *Visual*: Recall of visual representations.

16. What are the important brain structures for memory?

Ans. Two anatomic structures are of central importance in memory function.
- Medial portions of the dorsomedial nucleus of thalamus.
- Hippocampal formation of the medial temporal lobe.

17. What is the pathogenesis of transient global amnesia?

Ans. i. TGA is ischaemic or migrainous in nature.

ii. Bitemporal hypoperfusion is seen during an attack of TGA.

18. What is considered normal score in MMS?

Ans. A score of 24 or above in Mini Mental Scale of Folstein is considered normal.

19. How frequent are sleep disorders?

Ans. Sleep disorders are seen in 15 to 20% of adults.

20. What is polysomnography?

Ans. It is the continuous recording of the array of electro-physiologic parameters to define sleep and wakefulness.

21. What is the neural pacemaker for sleep?

Ans. Suprachiasmatic nuclei (SCN) of the hypothalamus.

22. What is melatonin?

Ans. i. The pineal hormone melatonin is secreted predominantly at night.

ii. The efficacy of melatonin as a sleep promoting therapy for patients with insomnia is currently not known.

23. What is REM sleep?

Ans. i. REM sleep seems to be the most important part of the sleep cycle for refreshing cognitive process.

ii. Dreams take place during REM sleep.

iii. REM sleep is associated with complete absence of thermo-regulatory responsiveness effectively resulting in functional poikilothermy.

24. What is narcolepsy?

Ans. Recurrent bouts of irresistible sleep are experienced during which the EEG often shows direct entry into REM sleep.

25. What is narcolepsy tetrad?

Ans. 1. Excessive daytime somnolence.

2. Cataplexy (sudden weakness or loss of muscle tone without loss of consciousness often elicited by emotion)

3. Hypnagogic hallucinations (hallucinations at sleep onset) and

   Hypnopompic hallucinations (hallucinations upon awakening)

4. **Sleep paralysis:** Muscle paralysis upon awakening.

26. What is the diagnosis of narcolepsy?

Ans. i. MSLT (multiple sleep latency test) less than 8 minutes.

ii. **Peptide hypocretin controls sleep:** A reduced level (below 110 pg/ml) of hypocretin in the spinal fluid is virtually diagnostic of narcolepsy.

27. What is the treatment of narcolepsy?

Ans. i. Modanafil (somnolence is treated with wake-promoting therapeutics) is given as 200 to 400 mg daily single dose.

ii. Tricyclic anti-depressants (protryptiline 10–40 mg per day)

Treatment of REM related phenomenon cataplexy, hypna-gogic hallucination and sleep paralysis requires the potent REM sleep suppression produced by anti-depressant medication.

28. What is the treatment of restless leg syndrome?

Ans. *Clonazepam*: 0.5 to 2 mg.

29. What is the treatment of periodic limb movement?

Ans. *Levodopa*: 100 to 200 mg HS.

30. What is parasomnia?

Ans. i. Parasomnias refer to abnormal behaviors that arise from or occur during sleep.

ii. Parasomnias occur during NREM sleep except REM sleep behavior disorder which occurs during REM sleep.

31. Discuss various parasomnias.

Ans. The distinctive feature of parasomnias is their occurrence only during sleep.

a. Sleep walking (somnambulism)

b. Sleep tremors

c. REM sleep behavior disorder

One third of patients will go onto develop Parkinson's disease within 10 to 20 years.

Treatment: Clonazepam 0.5 to 1 mg HS.

d. Sleep bruxism

Treatment: Benzodiazepines.

- **Sleep enuresis:** Normal feature before 5 years

Treatment: Imipramine 10 to 50 mg HS

- Nocturnal head banging (jactatio capitis nocturna).

32. What are circadian rhythm sleep disorders?

Ans. A subset of patients presenting with either insomnia or hypersomnia may have a disorder of sleep timing rather than sleep generation.

i. Rapid time zone change (jet-lag) syndrome

Treatment: Melatonin

ii. Shift work sleep disorder

iii. Delayed sleep phase syndrome

iv. Advanced sleep phase syndrome

v. Non 24 hours sleep wake disorders

Treatment: Melatonin low dose (0.5 mg).

33. What is the medical implication of circadian rhythmicity?

Ans. Platelet aggregability is increased after arising in the early morning hours, coincident with the peak incidence of the cardiovascular events.

34. What are sleep spindles?

Ans. On EEG, ½ to 2 seconds bursts of biparietal 12–14 hertz waves.

35. What are vertex waves (K complexes)?

Ans. Intermittent high—amplitude, central-parietal sharp slow, wave complexes.

36. What modulates or enhances dreams?

Ans. i. Dopaminergic systems in the basal forebrain elicit or modulate dreaming.

ii. There is enhancement of dreaming reported by patients taking L-dopa.

iii. According to Freud—in the book "the interpretation of dreams"—dreams express latent wishes and drives.

37. What happens to eastbound travellers?

Ans. They fall asleep late and face an early sunrise.

38. What is Kleine-Levin syndrome?

Ans. i. Kleine-Levin syndrome characterized by somnolence and overeating.

ii. **Lesion:** Medial thalamus and hypothalamus.

39. Describe the types of apnoea.

Ans. i. Central sleep apnoea (ondine's curse)
Treatment: Acetazolamide and oxygen
ii. Obstructive sleep apnoea
Treatment: CPAP (continuous positive airway pressure).

40. What is the treatment of nocturnal enuresis?

Ans. *Treatment*: Imipramine 10 to 75 mg at bedtime.
Nasal spray of anti-diuretic hormone (desmopressin) at bedtime.

41. What is mind?

Ans. It is a continuous inner consciousness of one's self and one's past experiences and ongoing cognitive activities.

42. What is confusion?

Ans. The patient's incapacity to think with customary speed, clarity and coherence is confusion.

43. What is amentia?

Ans. Amentia is a congenital feeble mindedness more commonly referred to mental retardation.

44. What is perception?

Ans. Perception is awareness.

45. What is apperception?

Ans. Interpretation of sensory stimuli is apperception.

46. What is confabulation?

Ans. Fabrication of stories is confabulation.

47. What is delusion?

Ans. When a false belief is maintained inspite of convincing evidence to the contrary, it is known as delusion.

48. What is mood?

Ans. Mood is prevailing emotional state of an individual without reference to the stimuli impinging upon him.

49. What is effect or feeling?

Ans. Effect or feeling refers to emotional reactions evoked by a thought or an environmental stimulus.

50. What is catatonia?

Ans. Catatonia is the condition when patient sits or lies silent and motionless with a staring countenance completely volition and reaction to sensory impressions.

51. What is akathesia?

Ans. Constant restless movements and inability to sit still is called akathesia.

52. What is beclouded dementia?

Ans. Dementia with superimposed acute confusional state or psychosis is beclouded dementia.

53. What is mesocortex?

Ans. The cortex of the cingulated gyrus which forms the outer ring of the limbic lobe, is transitional between neocortex and allocortex.

54. What is papez circuit?

Ans.

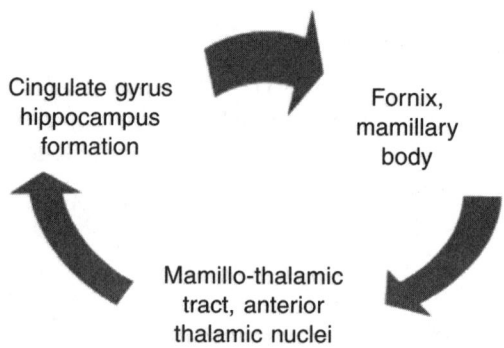

Cingulate gyrus hippocampus formation

Fornix, mamillary body

Mamillo-thalamic tract, anterior thalamic nuclei

55. Where is the zinc content highest in the nervous system?

Ans. Zinc content of the limbic system is the highest of any part of the nervous system.

56. What is pseudobulbar state in pseudobulbar palsy?

Ans. In this state, there is often a striking incongruity between the loss of voluntary movements of muscles innervated by the motor nuclei of the lower pons and medulla and the preservation of movement of the same muscles in yawning, coughing, spasmodic crying or laughing (reflexive pronto-medullary activities).

57. What is emotional lability?

Ans. In pseudobulbar, effective state on the slightest provocation and sometimes for no apparent reason, the patient laughs or cries. This is known as emotional lability.

58. What causes hypersexuality?

Ans. Superior frontal lesion causes hypersexuality.

59. What are the commonest causes of disinhibited sexual behaviour?

Ans. The commonest causes of disinhibited sexual behaviour are:
- Head injury
- Cerebral haemorrhage
- Dopaminergic drugs in Parkinson's disease.

60. What is Yerkes-Dodson law?

Ans. As anxiety increases, so does the standard of performance, but only to a point, after which increasing anxiety causes a rapid decline in performance. This is known as Yerkes-Dodson law.

11 Special Senses and Related Disorders

1. What are the unique features of olfactory nerve?

Ans. i. This the only site in the organism where neurons are in direct contact with the external environment.

ii. Olfactory impulses reach the cerebral cortex without relay through the thalamus. In this respect also, olfaction is unique among sensory systems.

iii. The olfactory receptor cells are constantly dying and being replaced by new ones. In this respect, the chemo-receptors, both for smell and taste are unique constituting the best defined example of neuronal regeneration in humans.

2. What are the important causes of anosmia?

Ans. i. Viral infections of the upper respiratory tract (largest group)

ii. Nasal or paranasal sinus disease

iii. Head injury

Smoking: It is probably the most frequent cause of hyposmia in clinical practice.

3. What is the cause of congenital anosmia?

Ans. Kallman syndrome is the cause of congenital anosmia.

4. What is the neoplastic cause of anosmia?

Ans. Meningioma of the inferior frontal region is the most frequent neoplastic cause of anosmia.

5. What are the taste sensations?

Ans. The sensations of taste are carried by:
- Salty
- Sweet
- Bitter
- Sour
- *Umani*: The taste of glutamate, aspartate and certain ribonucleotides has been added.

6. How are the sensations of taste carried?

Ans.
- *7th nerve*: Anterior two-thirds of the tongue
- *9th nerve*: Posterior one-thirds of the tongue
- *10th nerve*: Taste afferents from the larynx.

7. What are the important causes of taste dysfunction?

Ans. A side-effect of medication and smoking are the important causes of taste dysfunction.

8. What is the treatment of ageusia (loss of taste)?

Ans. Ageusia may respond to zinc.

9. What is amaurosis?

Ans. It refers to blindness, specifically blindness that is not due to intrinsic disease of the eye itself.

10. What is amblyopia?

Ans. It denotes a reduction of vision from any cause—ocular or non-ocular.

11. What is nyctalopia?

Ans. It is the term for poor twilight or night vision and is associated with
- i. Extreme myopia
- ii. Cataract
- iii. Vitamin A deficiency
- iv. Retinitis pigmentosa
- v. Colour blindness.

12. Why is lateral geniculate body of thalamus rarely infarcted?

Ans. The vascular supply of the lateral geniculate body is from both the posterior and anterior choridal and thalamo-geniculate arteries. It is therefore rarely infarcted.

13. What is the vascular supply of the eye?

Ans. Central retinal artery which is a branch of ophthalmic division of internal carotid artery.

14. What is the normal blind spot?

Ans. The absence of receptive elements in the optic disc or papilla account for the normal blind spot.

15. Where does the optic nerve get myelinated?

Ans. The ganglion-cell axon normally acquires their myelin sheath after penetration of the lamina cribrosa.

16. What are the hypertensive and arteriosclerotic changes of the retina?

Ans. Straightening of the arterioles and arteriovenous compression are the signs of hypertension and arteriosclerosis.

17. Discuss retinal haemorrhage.

Ans. a. *Splinter haemorrhage*: Occurs in superficial layers of the retina.

b. *Dot and blot haemorrhage*: Lies in synaptic layers between bipolar cells and rods and cones.

c. *Subhyaloid and preretinal haemorrhage*: Subarachnoid haemorrhage.

18. What are soft exudates or cotton wool patches?

Ans. They are in reality infarcts of the nerve fibre layer due to occlusion of precapillary arterioles. If present in the macular region, they are arranged in lines radiating towards the fovea called macular star.

19. What are hard exudates?

Ans. They consist of lipid and other serum precipitants due to abnormal vascular permeability of a type that is not completely understood.

Examples: Diabetes mellitus and chronic hypertension.

20. What is the characteristic finding of retina in infective endocarditis?

Ans. Roth's spots.

21. What is the pathogenesis of microaneurysms in DM?

Ans. Elevated levels of vascular endothelial growth factor have been shown to be the cause of retinal neovascularisation in diabetic retinopathy.

22. What is amaurosis fugax or transient monocular blindness (TMB)?

Ans. TMB is transient ischaemic attacks of visual loss involving all or part of the field of vision of one eye. They are common manifestations of atherosclerotic carotid stenosis or ulceration.

23. What are the features of central retinal artery occlusion?

Ans. The retina becomes opaque and have a gray-yellow appearance, the arterioles are narrowed with segmentation of volume of blood and a cherry-red appearance of fovea.

24. What are the features of thrombosis of the retinal vein?

Ans. i. Since the central retinal artery and vein share a common adventitial sheath, atheromatous plaques in the artery are said to be associated in some instances with the thrombosis of the retinal vein.

ii. There is a spectacular display of retinal lesions.

iii. The veins are engorged and tortuous and there are diffused dots and blots and streaky retinal haemorrhage.

25. What conditions cause retinal degeneration?

Ans. Retinitis pigmentosa and vigabatrin cause retinal degeneration.

26. What is the macular photostress test?

Ans. This test consists of shining a strong light through the pupil of an affected eye for 10 seconds and measuring the time necessary for the acuity to return to the pre-test level (normally 50 seconds or less). With macular lesions, recovery time is prolonged but with lesions of the optic nerve, it is not affected. This phenomenon may be observed in the eye on the side of the carotid occlusion, in essence an ischaemic retinopathy.

27. Discuss papilledema.

Ans.
  i. Presence of spontaneous venous pulsations is a reliable indicator of an intracranial pressure below 180 to 190 mm H_2O and thus excludes the presence of early papilledema.

  ii. Papilledema connotes bilateral optic disc swelling from raised intracranial pressure.

  iii. Transient visual obscurations are a classic symptom of papilledema.

  iv. Visual acuity is not affected by papilledema unless the papilledema is severe, long-standing or accompanied by macular edema and haemorrhage.

  v. Visual field testing shows enlarged blind spot and peripheral constriction.

  vi. The essential element in the pathogenesis of papilledema is an increase in pressure in the sheaths of the optic nerve which communicates directly with the subarachnoid space of the brain.

  vii. The pathogenesis of papilledema has also been ascribed to a blockage of axoplasmic flow in the optic nerve fibers.

  viii. With progression of the disease, reduction of optic disc swelling is an ominous sign of a dying nerve rather than an encouraging indication of a resolving papilledema.

28. What is Foster Kennedy syndrome?

Ans.
  i. The occurrence of papilledema on one side and optic atrophy on the other.

  ii. It is attributable to a frontal lobe tumor or olfactory meningioma on the side of the optic disc.

29. What is idiopathic intracranial hypertension?

Ans. i. An elevated pressure with normal cerebrospinal fluid points by exclusion to the diagnosis of psuedotumor cerebri (idiopathic intracranial hypertension).

ii. Treatment with a carbonic anhydrase inhibitor such as acetazolamide lowers intracranial pressure by reducing the production of CSF.

30. What is optic atrophy?

Ans. Loss of nerve fibres causes the optic disc to appear pale as the choroid becomes visible.

31. What are the hypertensive retinopathy changes?

Ans. *Cotton wool spots*: Focal infarcts of the nerve fibre layer
Hard exudates: Leakage of lipid and fluid.

32. What are the causes of blindness in diabetic retinopathy?

Ans. In advanced diabetic retinopathy, the proliferation of neovascular vessels leads to blindness from

i. Vitreous haemorrhage

ii. Retinal detachment

iii. Glaucoma.

33. What is the function of rods and cones?

Ans. There are 100 million rods and 5 million cones.
Functions:
Rods: They operate in dim vision (scotopic illumination).
Cones: They operate in daylight (photopic conditions).

34. Describe cone system.

Ans. i. The cone system is specialized for colour perception and high spatial resolution.

ii. The majority of cones are located within the macula, the portion of the retina serving the central 10° of vision.

iii. In the middle of the macula, a small pit termed as the fovea packed exclusively with cone, provides the best visual acuity.

35. Can diabetes cause myopia?

Ans. Yes, acute onset of DM can produce sudden myopia because of lens edema induced by hyperglycemia.

36. What are the primary colours?

Ans. i. Red x-linked ⎫
ii. Green ⎬
iii. **Blue:** Chromosome 7.

37. What are the causes of acquired colour blindness?

Ans. Disease of the:
- Optic nerve
- Macula
- Occipital cortex.

38. What are the causes of blindness from keratitis?

Ans. i. Trachoma from chlamydeal infection
ii. Vitamin A deficiency related to malnutrition.

39. What is the pathognomonic feature of herpes simplex?

Ans. A dendritic pattern of corneal epithelial ulceration is pathognomonic feature of herpes simplex.

40. What is Marcus Gunn Pupil?

Ans. i. If the retina or optic nerve has only partially injured the direct papillary, response will be weaker than the consensual papillary response evoked by shining a light into the other eye.
ii. This relative afferent papillary defect (Marcus Gunn Pupil) can be elicited with the swinging flashlight test.
iii. It is an extremely useful sign in retrobulbar optic neuritis and other optic nerve disease, where it may be the sole objective of the disease.

41. What is anisocoria?

Ans. Anisocoria is inequality in pupil size.

42. What is the relationship of sympathetic and parasympathetic lesion to anisocoria?

Ans. i. Anisocoria that increases in dim light indicates a sympathetic paresis of the iris dilator muscle.

ii. Anisocoria that increases in bright light suggests a parasympathetic palsy.

43. What is Horner's syndrome?

Ans. It is a triad of:

- Miosis
- Ipsilateral ptosis
- Anhidrosis

Etiology may be:

i. Brain stem stroke

ii. Carotid dissection

iii. Neoplasm, idiopathic.

44. What is Adie's syndrome?

Ans. i. *Tonic pupil*:

a. After denervation of the iris sphincter (parasympathetic paresis), the pupil does not respond well to light but the response to near is often really intact.

b. When the near stimulus is removed, the pupil redilates very slowly as compared with the normal pupil.

ii. *Adie's syndrome*:

a. In Adie's syndrome, a tonic pupil occurs in conjunction with weak or absent tendon reflexes in the lower extremity.

b. It is seen in dysautonomia (mild).

c. Denervation hypersensitivity to pilocarpine produces papillary constriction in a tonic pupil.

45. Describe field defects.

Ans. i. *Central*: Optic neuritis

ii. *Altitudinal*: Ischaemic neuropathy

iii. *Concentric constriction with enlargement of blind spot*: Papilledema

iv. *Scotoma*: An island of impaired vision surrounded by normal vision

v. *Junctional scotoma*: A scotomatous defect on the affected side coupled with a contralateral superior quadrantanopia (lesion is in Willibrand's knee)

vi. *Congruous field defects*: Occipital lobe

Incongruous field defects: Optic tract and optic radiations

vii. *Inferior quadrantanopia*: Though parietal lobe defects produce inferior quadrantanopia, it is difficult to document because in lesions of the right parietal lobe, the patient ignores the left half of the space and in left parietal lobe, the patient is often aphasic.

viii. *Superior quadrantanopia*: Temporal lobe lesions.

ix. *Homonymous altitudinal hemianopia*: Due to lesions of both occipital lobes below or above the calcarine sulcus.

46. What is visual agnosia?

Ans. The patient cannot understand the meaning of what he sees.

47. What is simultanagnosia?

Ans. Failure to understand the meaning of an entire picture even though some of its parts are recognized.

48. What is prosopagnosia?

Ans. Failure to recognize familiar faces is prosopagnosia.

49. What is palinopsia?

Ans. It is a persistence of repetitive after image. It occurs with right parieto-occipital lesion.

50. What are the complementary colours?

Ans. There are two pairs of complementary colours:
Red-green: Congenital, affected in optic nerve lesion
Yellow-blue: Affected in retinal lesion.

51. What are visual hallucinations?

Ans. There are two types:

   i. *Unformed simple visual hallucinations in epilepsy*: Due to stimulation of cortical termination

   ii. *Formed or complex visual hallucinations (people, animal, landscape)*: Due to diencephalon (peduncular hallucinosis).

52. What is visual allesthesia?

Ans. Patients in whom a hemianopia is evident only when tested by double simultaneous stimulation (attention hemianopia) may displace an image to the non-affected half of the field of vision.

53. What are saccades?

Ans.   i. Their purpose is to quickly change ocular fixation to bring images of new objects of interest onto the fovea.

   ii. Saccadic latency is approximately 200 milli seconds.

   iii. They are initiated in area 8 of the frontal lobe.

   iv. Peak velocity may exceed 700 degrees per second.

54. What are pursuit or following movements?

Ans.   i. The function of pursuit movements is to stabilize the image of a moving object on the fovea.

   ii. The major stimulus is a moving target.

   iii. They are generated in the ipsilateral parieto-occipital cortex.

55. What is opto-kinetic nystagmus?

Ans. Repeated cycles of pursuit and refixation.

56. What is vestibulo-ocular reflex?

Ans. A movement of the eye is produced that is equal and opposite to the movement of the head.

57. What is PPRF (Paramedian Pontine Reticular Formation)?

Ans. It is the pontine centre for horizontal gaze where ultimately all the pathways mediating saccadic and pursuit movements in the horizontal plane as well as vestibular and opto-kinetic movements converge.

58. Can gaze palsy cause diplopia?

Ans. No, cerebral gaze paralysis is not attended by diplopia because eyes move conjugately.

59. What lesions produce gaze-paretic nystagmus?

Ans. Cerebellar (floccular) lesion and PPRF produce gaze-paretic nystagmus.

60. What is Skew deviation?

Ans. Skew deviation is the vertical deviation of one eye above the other. Its causes are:

a. Brain stem and

b. Cerebellum.

61. What are the peculiarities of the innervations of infranuclear eye movements?

Ans. i. The superior rectus receives only crossed fibres.

ii. The levator palpebrae superioris has a bilateral innervation.

iii. Trochlear nerve innervates the contralateral superior oblique muscle.

62. What is the differentiating point between the anterior and posterior portions of cavernous sinus involvement?

Ans. i. In the anterior portion, only the ophthalmic division is affected.

ii. In the posterior portion, the first and second divisions of trigeminal nerve tend to be involved along with oculo-motor nerve.

63. What are the rules of diplopia?

Ans. i. The direction in which the images are maximally separated indicates the direction of action of a pair of muscles at fault.

ii. In the position of maximal separation, the image projected farther from the centre is attributable to the paretic muscle.

64. What is Tolosa-Hunt syndrome?

Ans. It is an idiopathic granulomatous condition.
Treatment: Steroids (prednisolone 60 mg and then tapered).

65. What is Duane-retraction syndrome?

Ans. Co-contraction of the medial and lateral recti results in retraction of the globe in all directions of ocular movement.

66. What is INO (inter nuclear opthalmoplegia)?

Ans. i. Adduction on the same side is affected due to MLF.
ii. Abducting eye has nystagmus due to Hering's law.

67. What is Hering's law?

Ans. When activated pairs of yoked muscles receives equal and simultaneous innervation because of an adaptive increase in innervations of the weak adductor, a commensurate increase in the innervations to the strong abductor occurs (manifest as a nystagmus), it is known as Hering's law.

68. Can MLF (median longitudinal fasciculus) cause skew?

Ans. i. Yes.
ii. MLF also contains axons that originate in the vestibular nuclei and govern vertical eye position and therefore can cause skew.

69. What is anterior INO?

Ans. High midbrain lesion may be associated with loss of convergence.

70. What is posterior INO?

Ans. A lesion in the pons where convergence is spared but horizontal gaze may be affected due to adjacent horizontal gaze centre.

71. What is one and half syndrome?

Ans. Pontine centre for gaze plus adjacent ipsilateral MLF getting affected produces only one and half movements.

72. What is top of the basilar syndrome?

Ans. It is the upgaze or complete vertical gaze palsy with psuedo-abducens palsy.

73. What is upside down vision?

Ans. i. Impaired vestibular-otolith nucleus.
  ii. Lateral medullary infarction is the most common cause.

74. What are the siginificant points of oculomotor nerve involvement?

Ans. i. The third nerve can get affected in posterior communicating artery aneurysm where pupil gets dilated.
  ii. Lesions of the oculomotor nucleus
  a. Bilateral ptosis because the levator muscle is innervated by a single central subnucleus.
  b. Weakness of the contralateral superior rectus because it is supplied by the oculomotor nucleus on the other side.
  c. Midbrain lesions cause
  • *Nothnagel's syndrome*: Injury to the superior cerebellar peduncle causes ipsilateral oculomotor palsy and contralateral cerebellar ataxia.
  • *Benedict's syndrome*: Injury to the red nucleus results in the ipsilateral oculomotor palsy and contralateral tremor, chorea and athetosis.
  • *Claude's syndrome*: Benedict's plus Nothnagel's (red nucleus plus superior cerebellar lesion).
  • *Weber's syndrome*: Injury to the cerebral peduncle causes ipsilateral oculomotor palsy with contralateral hemiparesis.
  iii. A significant point is that aberrant regeneration of the 3rd nerve is seen in trauma and compression but not after microvascular infarct, e.g. DM.

75. What are the significant points of trochlear nerve?

Ans. i. Fibres exist the brain stem dorsally and cross to innervate the contralateral superior oblique.

ii. Causes of trochlear nerve palsy
- Idiopathic (microvascular infarct)
- Closed head trauma.

76. What is the important difference of a nuclear lesion and a nerve lesion of 6th nerve?

Ans. a. *Nuclear lesion*: A nuclear lesion has different consequences because the abducens nucleus contains interneurons that project via the MLF to the medial rectus subnucleus of the contralateral oculomotor complex. Therefore, an abducens nuclear lesion produces a complete lateral gaze palsy from the weakness of both the ipsilateral rectus and the contralateral medial rectus.

b. *Nerve lesion*: It has lateral rectus weakness only.

77. What are the various syndromes associated with sixth nerve involvement?

Ans. i. *Foville's syndrome*: It follows dorsal pontine injury. It includes lateral gaze palsy, ipsilateral facial palsy and contralateral hemiparesis.

ii. *Millard Gubler syndrome*: It follows ventral pontine injury. There is a lateral rectus weakness only instead of gaze palsy because the abducens fasciculus is involved rather than the nucleus. There are also ipsilateral facial palsy and contralateral hemiparesis.

iii. *Gradenigo's syndrome*: At the petrous apex mastoiditis can produce deafness, pain and ipsilateral abducens palsy.

78. What is the relationship of 6th nerve with raised intracranial pressure?

Ans. i. Unilateral or bilateral abducens palsy is a classic sign of raised intracranial pressure.

ii. The mechanism is related to the rostral-caudal displacement of the brain stem.

79. What are the causes of multiple ocular motor nerve palsies?

Ans. i. Diabetes mellitus
a. Microinfarcts of all nerves
b. Fungal infection (Aspergillus, Mucorales, Cryptococcus)

Note: Neuroimaging should focus on the cavernous sinus, superior orbital fissure and orbital apex where all the oculomotor nerves are in close proximity.

ii. Carcinomatous meningitis

iii. Lambert-eaten myasthenic syndrome

iv. Giant cell (temporal) arteritis

v. **Fisher syndrome:** An ocular variant of GBS can produce ophthalmoplegia with areflexia and ataxia. Antiganglioside antibodies (GQ1b) can be detected in about 50% of cases

80. What are the supranuclear disorders of gaze palsy?

Ans. i. Wernicke's encephalopathy

ii. Progressive supranuclear palsy.

81. How to differentiate between PPRF lesion and abducens nucleur lesion both of which cause horizontal gaze palsy?

Ans. Vestibular stimulation (oculocephalic maneuver or caloric irrigation) will succeed in driving the eyes conjugately to the side in a patient with a lesion of PPRF but not in a patient with a lesion of abducens nucleus.

82. What is Parinaud's syndrome?

Ans. It is a dorsal midbrain syndrome. It consists of:

- Loss of upgaze and sometimes downgaze
- Convergence-retraction nystagmus
- Setting sun sign
- Collier's sign (lid retraction)
- Skew deviation.

83. Describe nystagmus.

Ans. • Nystagmus refers to the involuntary rhythmic movements of the eye.

- **Types of nystagmus:**
  a. **Jerk nystagmus:** Alternating fast and slow components
  b. **Pendular nystagmus:** Oscillations are roughly equal in both directions.

- **Classification of nystagmus** (as a result of disturbance of):
  a. Vestibular apparatus or its brain stem nuclei
  b. **Cerebellum:** Gage evoked nystagmus is the most common form of jerk nystagmus.
  c. Number of specific regions of the brain stem such as MLF
  d. Drugs (sedatives, anti-convulsants, alcohol) intoxication is the most frequent cause of nystagmus.
  e. **Downbeat nystagmus:** It occurs from lesions near the craniocervical junction (e.g. chiari malformation).
  f. **Upbeat nystagmus:** It is associated with the damage to the pontine tegmentum form stroke, demyelination or tumour.
  g. **Miscellaneous:**
     i. Muscle paresis
     ii. Myasthenia gravis.

84. Describe nystagmus of labyrinthine origin.

Ans.　i. Tonic inputs from the vestibular apparatus project to the contralateral 6th nerve nucleus via the vestibular nucleus.

ii. In lesions of the vestibular system (most commonly peripheral labyrinthine lesion), damage to the horizontal canal or its connections on one side will allow the tonic output from the healthy contralateral side to cause the eyes to drift towards the side of the lesion.

iii. This causes recurrent compensatory fast movements away from the side of the lesion, hence unidirectional horizontal nystagmus to the opposite side is seen.

iv. **Alexander's law:** Vestibular nystagmus of peripheral (labyrinthine) origin in most cases beats away from the side of the lesion and increases as the eyes are turned in the direction of the quick phase.

v. Pure labyrinthine origin has a characteristically torsional component.

vi. Nystagmus is suppressed with visual fixation.

85. Describe nystagmus due to brain stem and cerebellar disease.

Ans. i. The brain stem and cerebellum are involved in maintaining eccentric position of the gaze.

ii. Lesions will therefore allow eyes to drift back in towards the primary position.

iii. This produces nystagmus whose fast component beats in the direction of the gaze.

iv. **Rebound nystagmus:** It is a gaze-evoked nystagmus that changes directions with refixation to the primary position. It is seen in vestibulocerebellar lesions.

v. Brain stem lesions often cause a course, unidirectional gaze dependent nystagmus.

86. What is dissociated nystagmus?

Ans. It is an abducting nystagmus. It is a common sign of internuclear ophthalmoplegia.

87. What is opsoclonus?

Ans. i. Seen in viral encephalitis

ii. *Saccadomania*: Bursts of consecutive saccades

iii. *Ocular flutter*: When the saccades are confined to the horizontal plane.

88. What is oscillopsia?

Ans. It is the illusory movement of the environment in which stationary objects seem to move back and forth. It is due to labyrinthine lesion and impaired VOR (vestibulo-oculo reflex) function.

89. What is pendular nystagmus?

Ans. i. This is found in a variety of conditions in which central vision is lost early in life such as albinism.

ii. *Miner's nystagmus*: An associated condition that occurs in patients who have worked for many years in comparative darkness.

iii. *Spasmus nutans*: Due to idiopathic/chiasmal/3rd ventricular tumour. It is a specific type of pendular nystagmus of infancy which is accompanied by head nodding and occasionally by wry neck.

90. What is optokinetic nystagmus?

Ans. i. When one is watching a moving object, a rhythmic jerk nystagmus (OKN) normally appears.

ii. With unilateral lesions of the parietal region, the slow phase of OKN is lost when the drum is rotated towards the side of the lesion.

iii. The presence of OKN proves that the patient is not blind.

iv. A nasal OKN is established within hours after birth.

91. What are the other various types of nystagmus?

Ans. i. *Convergence nystagmus*: It refers to a rhythmic oscillation in which a slow abduction of the eye in respect to each other is followed by a quick movement of adduction.

It is usually accompanied by quick rhythmic retraction movements of the eyes (nystagmus retractorius).

It is seen in parinaud-dorsal midbrain syndrome.

ii. *See-saw nystagmus*: Torsional-vertical oscillation in which the intorting eye moves up and opposite (extorting) eye moves down, then both move in reverse direction.

Lesion: Sellar or parasellar masses.

iii. *Periodic-alternating nystagmus*: Horizontal jerking that periodically (every 90 seconds or so) changes direction.

Lesion: Lower brain stem lesion, CJD diseases

iv. *Palatal nystagmus*: Central tegmental tract lesion.

92. What are the other spontaneous ocular movements?

Ans. i. *Ping-pong gaze*: Roving eye movements seen in bi-hemispheric infarctions.

ii. *Ocular bobbing*: Fast downward jerk of the eyes followed by a slow upward drift to the midposition with absence of horizontal eye movements.

For example, pontine lesion.

iii. *Ocular dipping*: Arrhythmic slow conjugate downward movement followed by a rapid upward movement.

For example, anoxic encephalopathy.

iv. *Saccadomania*:

- Rapid conjugate oscillations of the eye in horizontal rotatory and vertical direction.
- Saccadomania is unique among disorders of ocular movement in that they persist in sleep.
- Seen in: (a) Paraneoplastic manifestations with severe ataxia and (b) AIDS.

93. What are the disorders of the eyelids?

Ans. i. *Blinking*: It occurs irregularly at a rate of 12 to 20 per minute.

ii. A reduced frequency of blinking (<10 per minute) is seen in Parkinson's disease.

iii. *Myerson's sign*: The failure to inhibit this glabellar tap response.

iv. Aberrant 7th nerve regeneration

a. *Jaw-winking phenomenon*: Eyelid retracts when the mouth is opened.

b. *Inverse Marcus-Gunn phenomenon, Marin-Amat syndrome*: Eyelid closes when the mouth is opened.

v. Combined paralysis of the levator and orbicularis oculi muscles (muscles that open and close the lids) nearly always indicate a myopathic disease such as myasthenia gravis or myotonic dystrophy.

vi. Retraction of the upper lids (opposite of ptosis) is seen in thyroid disorder.

94. Discuss pupillary abnormalities.

Ans. i. *Marcus-Gunn pupillary sign*: Slowness of response along with failure to sustain papillary constriction.

ii. *Hippus*: A rapid alteration in pupillary sign is common in metabolic encephalopathy.

iii. *Ciliospinal pupillary reflex*: Stimulation of sympathetic fibres cause dilatation of the pupil. Ciliospinal reflex is evoked by pinching the neck (afferent C_2 C_3) and is affected through the efferent sympathetic fibres.

iv. *Miosis*: Commonly observed with pontine lesions because of bilateral interruption of pupillodilator fibers.

v. *Argyl-Robertson pupil*: It is a light near dissociation phenomenon. It is seen in
   • Late syphilis
   • DM
   • Lyme disease

vi. *Adie-tonic pupil (homes-adie syndrome)*:
   • Degeneration of ciliary ganglia and the postganglionic parasympathetic fibres that normally constrict the pupil and affect accommodation.
   • Constriction and redilatation occurs slowly.
   • Absence of knee and ankle jerks.
   • Denervation supersensitivity.

vii. *Springing pupil*: Transient episodes of unilateral mydriasis. Its causes are:
   a. Idiopathic
   b. Use of mydriatic solution in cardiac resuscitation

viii. *Anisocoria*: Unequal pupil
   a. Cocaine does not dilate the pupil of Horner's syndrome because of the absence of neurotransmitter.
   b. After confirmation of Horner's syndrome with cocaine if pupil does not dilate with 1% hydroxyamphetamine, it is postganglionic and vice versa.

95. What are the components of jaw jerk?

Ans. *Afferent*: Proprioceptive afferents that terminate in the mesencephalic nucleus.
Efferent: Collateral to the motor nucleus of 5th nerve and causes the masseter to contract.

96. What is the essential feature of trigeminal neuralgia?

Ans. An essential feature of trigeminal neuralgia is that objective signs of sensory loss cannot be demonstrated on examination.

97. What is the treatment of trigeminal neuralgia?

Ans. 1. Carbamazepine 200 mg qid
2. Radio frequency thermal rhizotomy
3. Microvascular decompression.

98. What is Ramsay-Hunt syndrome?

Ans. This syndrome is due to herpes zoster of the geniculate ganglion. It consists of a severe facial palsy associated with a vesicular eruption in the pharynx, external auditory canal.

99. What is Melkersson-Rosenthal syndrome?

Ans. This syndrome is a triad of:
i. Recurrent facial paralysis
ii. Facial particularly labial edema
iii. Plication of the tongue.

100. What are the causes of LMN facial paralysis?

Ans. i. Ramsay-Hunt syndrome.
ii. GBS
iii. Uveoparotid fever (Heerfordt syndrome), a form of sarcoidosis.

101. What is the treatment of Bell's palsy?

Ans. i. *Predniosolone*: 60 mg for 5 days and then tapered over 5 days (total 10 days)
ii. *Acyclovir*: 400 mg 5 times daily for 10 days.

102. What is the treatment of hemifacial spasm?

Ans. i. Carbamazepine
ii. Baclofen.

103. What is Fisher variant of GBS?

Ans. i. Oculomotor paresis
ii. Ataxia
iii. Areflexia.

104. What is Tolosa-Hunt syndrome?

Ans. i. Idiopathic granulomatous disorder

ii. Responds to glucocorticoids.

105. When should the treatment of Bell's palsy and GBS be intiated?

Ans. In Bell's palsy, steroids should be started within 3 days.

In GBS, immunoglobulins should be started within 14 days.

106. What are the poor prognostic factors in Bell's palsy and GBS?

Ans. i. *In Bell's palsy:*

• Complete paralysis

• Old age

• Reduced facial motor action potential amplitude after first week

ii. *In GBS:*

• Rapid deterioration to ventilation

• Old age

• Evidence of axonal loss on EMG.

107. What is Tullio's phenomenon?

Ans. Vertigo induced by loud, high pitched sounds or by yawning due to spontaneous or traumatic fenestration of the vestibule of the semicircular canal.

108. What is the frequency of hearing loss disorder?

Ans. Nearly 10% of the adult population has some hearing loss.

109. What causes conductive and sensori-neural hearing loss?

Ans. In general, lesions in the auricle, external auditory canal or middle ear causes conductive hearing loss whereas lesions in the inner ear or 8th nerve causes sensori-neural hearing loss.

110. What transduces linear and angular movement of the head? What are the systems which subserve spatial orientation?

Ans. The labyrinthine semi-circular canals transduce-angular movements of the head and the otoliths transducer linear movement.

The systems which subserve spatial orientation are:

- Vestibular system
- Visual system
- Somatosensory system.

111. What is the pattern in normal hearing and deafness disorders?

Ans. Normally, air conduction is better than bone conduction. Conductive deafness is characterized by a partial loss of low-pitched sounds and sensori-neural deafness is characterized by a partial loss of high pitched sounds.

112. What is recruitment and diplacusis?

Ans. *Recruitment*: It refers to a heightened perception of loudness once the threshold for hearing loss has been exceeded.

Diplacusis: Defect in frequency discrimination that is manifested by a lack of clarity of spoken syllables or by the perception that music is out of tune or unpleasant. (A cochlear type of hearing loss has recruitment and diplacusis.)

113. What is tinnitus?

Ans. It is any sensation of sound for which there is no source outside the individual. Aspirin can cause tinnitus.

114. What is paracusis?

Ans. It is a cerebral auditory phenomenon similar to visual phenomenon of palinopsia.

115. What is epileptic suppression of hearing?

Ans. A brief episode of deafness with fully preserved consciousness may rarely be caused by seizure activity in one temporal lobe.

116. What causes auditory hallucinosis?

Ans. Pontine lesions can cause pontine auditory hallucinosis.

117. What is the characteristic feature of labyrinthine and cerebellar disorders?

Ans. *Labyrinthine disorder*: Predominantly unidirectional nystagmus to the opposite side of the impaired labyrinth and swaying or falling towards the involved side.
Cerebellar disease: Falling and nystagmus are towards the lesion.

118. What is the most certain sign of a labyrinthine disorder?

Ans. Changing from a recumbent to a sitting position reverses the direction of vertigo and nystagmus.

119. What are the characteristic features of BPPV (benign paroxysmal positional vertigo)?

Ans. i. Elicitation by change in head position
ii. Latency of onset
iii. Reversal of direction of nystagmus on sitting up
iv. Fatigability with repetition of the test
v. Long and recurrent vertigo.

120. Differentiate between the nystagmus of brain stem and labyrinthine origins.

Ans. *Brain stem origin*:
- Uni or bidirectional
- Purely horizontal, vertical or rotatory
- Characteristically worsened by visual fixation
Labyrinthine origin:
- Unidirectional
- Usually with the rotatory component
- Past pointing and falling are in the direction of slow phase
- Purely vertical nystagmus does not occur
- Purely horizontal nystagmus without a rotatory component is unusual
- Inhibited by visual fixation
- Reverse direction with changes in position of the head.

12 Autonomic Nervous System and Related Conditions

1. What is postural hypotension?

Ans. Bedside testing of orthostatic blood pressure is best performed by having the patient stand quickly and taking readings immediately and again at 1 and 3 minutes.

Systolic difference of more than 20 mmHg and diastolic difference of more than 10 mmHg defines postural hypotension.

2. What is valsalva maneuver?

Ans. In the valsalva maneuver, the subject exhales into a manometer or against a closed glottis for 10 to 15, creating a markedly positive intrathoracic pressure. The sharp reduction in venous return to the heart causes a drop in cardiac output and in blood pressure; the response on baroreceptors is to cause a reflex tachycardia and to a lesser extent, peripheral vasoconstriction. With release of intrathoracic pressure, the venous return, stroke volume and blood pressure rise to higher than normal levels; reflex parasympathetic influences then predominates and a bradycardia results.

   i. Failure of the heart rate increase during the positive intrathoracic pressure phase of the valsalva maneuver that points to sympathetic dysfunction, and

   ii. Failure of the rate decrease during the period of blood pressure overshoot that points to a parasympathetic disturbance.

3. **What is valsalva ratio?**

Ans. Valsalva maneuver has four phases:
Phase I: Rise in BP
Phase II: Gradual fall in BP to plateau
Tachycardia (if not indicates sympathetic dysfunction)
Phase III: Fall in BP
Phase IV: Overshoot of BP
Bradycardia (if not indicates parasympathetic dysfunction)
Valsalva ratio is defined as the maximum phase II
tachycardia divided by the minimum phase IV bradycardia.

4. **When does autonomic dysfunction begin in diabetes?**

Ans. Autonomic neuropathy typically begins 10 years after the
onset of diabetes and slowly progresses.

5. **What is GIT autonomic dysfunction?**

Ans. Damage to the autonomic components usually causes
constipation but diabetic neuropathy may be associated with
diarrhea.

6. **Discuss neurogenic and non-neurogenic orthostatic hypotension.**

Ans. i. An important clue that the patient has neurogenic OH is
the aggravation or precipitation of OH by autonomic
stressors (such as a meal, hot bath and exercise).
ii. In non-neurogenic cause of OH (such as hypovolemia),
the BP drop is accompanied by a compensatory increase
in heart rate of more than 15 beats per minute.

7. **How much percentage of GBS patients suffer from cardiovascular collapse?**

Ans. 2–10%.

8. **What are the manifestations of impaired baroreflex?**

Ans. i. Supine hypertension
ii. Heart rate that is fixed regardless of posture
iii. Postprandial hypotension
iv. Excessive high nocturnal BP.

9. How does sympathetic nervous system originate?

Ans. The preganglionic neurons of the sympathetic division originate in the intermediolateral cell column of the spinal gray matter from the eighth cervical to the second lumbar segment.

10. What is uniqueness of adrenal medulla?

Ans. The sympathetic innervation of the adrenal medulla is unique in that its secretory cells receive preganglionic fibres directly via the splanchnic nerve.

This is an exception to the rule that organs innervated by the ANS receive only post-ganglionic fibres.

11. What is the central regulation of visceral functions?

Ans. *In the brain stem*: NTS (nucleus tractus solitarius)
In the cerebrum: Hypothalamus.

12. Where does the integration of ANS and endocrine system occur?

Ans. The integration of ANS and endocrine system is achieved primarily in hypothalamus.

13. What are the peculiar physiologic consideration of ANS?

Ans. i. *Some structures*: Sweat glands, cutaneous blood vessels and hair follicles receive only sympathetic postganglionic fibres.
 ii. Adrenal gland has only a preganglionic sympathetic innervation.

14. Discuss acetylcholine.

Ans. i. It is released at the terminals of all preganglionic fibres (in both sympathetic and parasympathetic ganglia).
 ii. It is also released at the terminals of all postganglionic parasympathetic fibres.
 iii. It is also released in a few special postganglionic sympathetic fibres mainly those subserving sweat glands.
 iv. Acetylcholine is also the chemical transmitter of nerve impulses to the skeletal muscle fibres.

15. What are acetylcholine receptors?

Ans. *Muscarinic*:
- They are located within the innervated organ
- They are antagonized by atropinic drugs.

Nicotonic:
- They are located in the ganglia and skeletal muscle
- They are not blocked by atropine but by tubocurarine.

16. Discuss adrenergic receptors.

Ans. *α receptors*: They mediate vasoconstriction, relaxation of the gut, dilation of the pupil.

Alpha$_1$ receptors are post-synaptic whereas $α_2$ receptors are situated on the presynaptic membrane and when stimulated diminish the release of the transmitter.

β receptors:
- *$β_1$ receptors*: Limited to the heart. Their activity increases the heart rate and contractility.
- *$β_2$ receptors*:
  - Relaxes the smooth muscles of the bronchi
  - Dilates the blood vessels of skeletal muscles.

17. What are baroreceptors?

Ans. i. They are pressure change responding receptors.
  ii. Carotid sinus ⎫ are sensitive to reduction in pulse pressure
  Aortic arch ⎭ (the difference in systolic and diastolic blood pressure).

18. What are volume change responders?

Ans. i. Right heart chamber ⎫ respond to alterations in blood.
  ii. Pulmonary vessels ⎭

19. What are the two-slower acting hormonal mechanisms that regulate blood volume?

Ans. i. Pressure sensitive renal juxtaglomerular cells release renin which affects an increase of blood volume.
  ii. Antidiuretic hormone.

20. What are the factors on which blood pressure is dependent?

Ans. i. Adequacy of intravascular blood volume

ii. Systemic vascular resistance

iii. Cardiac output.

21. Describe the tests for abnormalities of the ANS (autonomic nervous system)?

Ans. I. **Response of blood pressure and heart rate to changes in posture and breathing**

- *Postural hypotension (>20/10)*:

  a. Hypovolemia

  b. Inadequate sympathetic vasoconstrictor activity

- *Simplest bedside indicator of vagal nerve dysfunction*: The failure of the heart rate to rise in response to the drop in blood pressure with standing.

- 30:15 < 1.05 is abnormal.

- *Variation in heart beat during deep breathing*: (Difference of less than 10 beats per minute between expiration and inspiration is abnormal).

- *Expiratory/inspiratory ratio*: Up to age 40, less than 1.2 is abnormal. Beyond 60 less than 1.04 is abnormal.

- *Valsalva maneuver*.

II. **Tests of vasomotor reactions:** Measurement of the skin temperature is a useful index of vasomotor function. Vasomotor paralysis results in vasodilatation of skin vessels and a rise in skin temperature.

a. *Cold pressor test*: Vasoconstriction induces an elevation of blood pressure. In normal persons, immersing one hand in ice water for 1 to 5 minutes raises the systolic pressure by 15 to 20 mm of mercury and diastolic pressure by 10 to 15 mm of mercury.

b. *Sustained isometric contraction*: Sustained isometric contraction of a group of muscles (e.g. those of forearm in handgrip) for 5 minutes normally increases the heart rate and systolic and diastolic pressure by at least 15 mmHg.

The response in both of these tests is reduced or absent with lesions of efferent limb of the sympathetic reflex arc.

c. *Mental arithmetic test*: The stress involved in doing mental arithmetic in noisy and distracting surroundings will also stimulate a mild but measureable increase in pulse rate and blood pressure.

Interpretation:

- If the response to the valsalva maneuver is abnormal and the response to cold pressor test is normal, the lesion is probably in the baroreceptors or their afferent nerves. Such a defect has been found in diabetic and tabetic patients and is common in many neuropathies.

- A failure of the pulse rate and blood pressure to rise during mental arithmetic coupled with an abnormal valsalva maneuver suggests a defect in the central or peripheral efferent sympathetic pathways.

- **Tests of sudomotor function:**

  Principle: The change in electrical potential is the result of an ionic current within sweat glands, not simply an increase in sweating that lowers skin resistance.

  a. Sympathetic or galvanic skin-resistance test

  b. Postganglionic sudomotor function test (QSART).

- **Lacrimal function:**

  Schirmer test: Lacrimation and tearing is estimated roughly.

- *Tests of bladder, gastrointestinal and penile erection function*:

  a. Bladder function:
     - Assessed by cystometrogram
     - Measurement of residual urine

  b. Disorders of gastrointestinal motility:
     - Rapidly demonstrated radiographically
     - Sophisticated manometry techniques are now available for the measurement of gastrointestinal motility especially esophagus.

c. Nocturnal penile tumescence—is recorded in many sleep laps and may be used as an ancillary test of sacral autonomic (parasympathetic) innervation.

- **Pharmacological tests of autonomic function:** Cannon's law or the phenomenon of denervation hypersensitivity: In it, an effector organ 2 to 3 weeks after denervation becomes hypersensitive to its particular neurotransmitter substance and related drugs.
  a. Epinephrine instillation
     - No effect on normal pupil.
     - Will cause sympathetically denervated pupil to dilate. The hypersensitivity is greater with lesions of postganglionic fibres than of pre-ganglionic fibers.
  b. Coccaine
     - Dilates normal pupil
     - Coccine potentiates the effects of norepinephrine by preventing its uptake. In sympathetic denervation caused by lesions of post- or preganglionic fibres no change in pupillary size occurs, since no transmitter substance is available.
- **Cutaneous flare response to histamine:** It may be absent in peripheral neuropathies that involve sympathetic nerves. Examples are
  - Diabetes
  - Alcohol-nutritional disease
  - GB syndrome
  - Amyloidosis
  - Porphyria
- **Pressor infusion and other direct cardiovascular tests:**
  a. Norepinephrine and angiotensin II cause a rise in blood pressure which is usually more pronounced for a given infusion rate in dysautonomic states, e.g. GB syndrome than it is with normal subjects.
     Explanation:
     - Defective baroreceptor function
     - Denervation hypersensitivity.

    b. Atropine does not increase heart rate in:

      a. DM

      b. GBS.

      c. Brain death

    c. Norepinephrine level rises two to three-fold from supine to standing normally.

22. What are the bedside tests of ANS?

Ans.   i. Measurement of orthostatic pulse and BP changes.

    ii. Blood pressure response to valsalva maneuver.

    iii. Estimation of pulse changes with deep breathing.

    iv. Pupillary response to light and dark.

    v. Rough estimate of sweating of palms and soles.

23. Discuss clinical disorders of ANS.

Ans.   i. Acute autonomic paralysis

    ii. Primary autonomic failure, idiopathic orthostatic hypotension

     Treatment:

      • Fludocortisone 0.1 mg twice daily.

      • Elastic stockings compresses the veins of the legs and lower abdomen.

    iii. Peripheral neuropathy with secondary orthostatic hypotension

      • Diabetic neuropathy

      • Amyloid neuropathy

    iv. Autonomic neuropathy in infants and children

      • Riley-Day syndrome

      • Fabry disease

    v. Autonomic neuropathy in elderly

    vi. Horner's syndrome

     Ross syndrome: The combination of segmental anhidrosis and an adie pupil.

    vii. Sympathetic and parasympathetic paralysis in tetraplegia and paraplegia.

viii. *Mass reflex*: Flexor spasms of the legs and involuntary emptying of the bladder are associated with a marked rise in blood pressure, bradycardia and sweating and pilomotor reactions in parts below the cervical segments (autonomic dysreflexia).

ix. *Acute autonomic crises (sympathetic storm)*:
- *Cocaine*: Abrupt hypersensitivity of sympathetic and parasympathetic nervous system
- *Tricyclic anti-depressants*: Cholinergic blockade
- *Organophosphate insecticides*: Parasympathetic over activity and motor paralysis
- *Tetanus*: Circulatory catecholamines
- Severe head injury and intracerebral haemorrhage (*three stages*):

  Ist stage: An acute outpouring of adrenal catecholamines at the time of ictus with acute hypertension and tachycardia.

  IInd stage: Cushing response (a brain stem mediated vasopressor response)

  As a result of an abrupt increase in intracranial pressure, it consists of a triad of:
  - Hypertension
  - Bradycardia
  - Slow irregular breathing

  IIIrd stage: Diencephalic autonomic seizures

  Extreme hypertension, profuse diaphoresis and pupillary dilatation usually arising during episodes of several minutes duration of rigid extensor posturing.

24. Discuss disorders of sweating.

Ans.
i. Hyperhidrosis: It results from over activity of sudomotor nerve fibres under a variety of conditions.
ii. Horner's syndrome does not develop if T_1 ganglion is left intact.
iii. Sweating is not affected in spinal root disease because there is much intersegmental mixing of the pre-ganglionic axons once they enter the sympathetic chain.

Raynaud syndrome: This disorder is characterized by
- Painful blanching of the fingers
- Presumably caused by digital artery spasm
- Episodes are brought on by cold and emotional stress and usually followed by redness on rewarming.

Raynaud disease: Idiopathic

Raynaud phenomenon: Secondary to connective tissue disorders (scleroderma)

Pathogenesis:
- Arterial constriction
- Decrease in intraluminal pressure

Treatment:
1. Avoidance of cold exposure drugs that cause vaso-constriction.
2. Calcium channel blockers: Nifedipine 30 to 60 mg per day.

25. Discuss disturbances of bladder function.

Ans. Multiple sclerosis usually with uneasy urgency is by far the most common neurologic disorder that causes bladder dysfunction.

Lesions of bladder function:
  i. *Complete destruction of the cord below T_{12} and conus*: Voiding is possible only by Crede maneuver.
  ii. Diseases of the sacral motor neurons in the spinal gray matter, the anterior sacral roots or peripheral nerves innervating the bladder.
  iii. Interruption of the sensory afferent fibres.
  iv. Reflexive neurogenic spastic bladder (upper spinal cord lesion above T_{12}).

Common causes:
- Multiple sclerosis
- Traumatic myelopathy
- Myelitis
- Spondylosis
- AVM
- Syringomyelia

- Tropical spastic paraparesis
- Mixed type of neurogenic bladder
- Stretch injury of the bladder wall
- Frontal lobe incontinence
- Nocturnal enuresis or urinary incontinence during sleep.

Treatment:
- Flaccid paralysis: Bethanchol (urecholine)
- Spastic paralysis:
  a. Propanthelene 15 to 30 mg three times daily
  b. Oxybutinin 5 mg two or three times daily
- Alpha 1 sympathetic blockers (terazosin). Releases the urinary sphincter and facilitates voiding.

Uses:
- Prostatic hypertrophy
- Dextrusor sphincter dyssynergia.

26. Discuss disturbance of bowel function.

Ans. Disturbance of bowel function refers to
- Anismus (severe constipation)
- *Myasthenia*: Early sign → An inability to control flatulence.

27. What is impotence?

Ans. Sexual desire may be present but penile erection is impossible to attain or sustain.

Causes:
- Depressive state
- Prostatectomy
- Diseases of the spinal cord
  - Tumour, myelitis, tabes
- Diabetes and other peripheral neuropathies.

28. What is the nervous system control of respiration?

Ans. 1. Pre-botzinger area in the medulla may play a special role in generating the respiratory rhythm.
2. Dorsal respiratory group (DRG) contains inspiratory neurons.
3. Ventral respiratory group (VRG) contains expiratory neurons.

4. Pontine Pair of Nuclei (PRG) one of which fires in the transition between inspiration and expiration and the other between expiration and inspiration.

29. Why tonicity does not affect diaphragm?

Ans. Diaphragm is not subject to spasticity with cortico spinal lesion because it has a paucity of spindle receptors when compared with other skeletal muscles (a property shared with extraocular muscles) and to the loss of tone in states such as REM sleep in which gamma motor neurons are greatly diminished.

30. What is Ondine's curse?

Ans. Loss of automatic respiration during sleep with preserved voluntary breathing and therefore requires CPAP during night.

31. What is effective in hiccup (Singultus)?

Ans. Baclofen is sometimes effective.

32. What are the disorders of ventilation due to neuromuscular diseases?

Ans. *Acute causes*:
* GBS
* Myasthenia gravis

Sub-acute or chronic causes:
* Motor neuron disease
* Myopathies (acid maltase, nemaline)
* Muscular dystrophies.

33. What is the normal breathing rate?

Ans. Normal breathing rate is 16 per minute.

34. Discuss neurologic basis of swallowing.

Ans. i. Swallowing occurs at a nocturnal frequency of about once per minute.

ii. Unlike the generators of respiratory rhythm, the entire reflex apparatus for swallowing may be located in the NTS.

iii. Sometimes recurrent minor pneumonias are the only manifestations of intermittent (silent) aspiration.

iv. Dysphagia:

a. *Defect in the initiation of swallowing*: There is usually an associated dysarthria with difficulty in pronouncing lingual sounds.

Causes:
- Myasthenia gravis
- Motor neuron disease
- Inflammatory disease of the muscle
- 12th nerve palsy

b. *Second type of dysphagia is associated with nasal regurgitation*: A nasal pattern of speech with air escaping from the nose is a usual accompaniment.

Casues:
- Myasthenia gravis
- 10th nerve palsy
- Incoordination of swallowing due to bulbar or psuedobulbar palsy.

35. What is melatonin?

Ans. It is a pineal hormone. Its cyclic secretion maintains biologic (circadian) rhythm.

36. What causes diabetes insipidus?

Ans. 1. Carbamazepine
2. Lithium.

37. What is blood osmolality? What is osmotic threshold?

Ans. *Blood osmolality*: 282 m mol/kg
Osmotic threshold: 287 m mol/kg (release of ADH begins).

38. What is neurogenic (cerebral) salt wasting?

Ans. It is due to atrial natriuretic factor (ANF).

39. What is Fröhlich's syndrome?

Ans. It is adiposogenital dystrophy.

Pituitary tumour causes:
a. Obesity
b. Gonadal underdevelopment.

40. What are the appetite and satiety centers in hypothalamus?

Ans. *Appetite center*: Ventrolateral nucleus of hypothalamus
Satiety center: Ventromedian nucleus of hypothalamus.

41. What causes hyperthermia?

Ans. Bilateral lesions in the anterior parts of hypothalamus causes hyperthermia.

42. What is the mechanism of cardiovascular disorders with hypothalamic lesions?

Ans. Hypothalamus mounting a massive sympathoadrenal discharge is the likely source of cardiovascular changes.

43. What is cushing ulcer?

Ans. Superficial erosions or ulceration of the gastric mucosa in the absence of hyperacidity due to lesions in the tuberal nuclei is known as cushing ulcer.

44. What is neurogenic pulmonary edema?

Ans. Without obvious left ventricular failure, hypothalamus may
  • Exert a direct sympathetic influence on the pulmonary vasculature allowing a leakage of protein rich edema fluid.
  • Edema may be the result of sudden and massive over-loading of pulmonary vasculature by a shift of fluid from the systemic vasculature.

45. What lesions are associated with stupor?

Ans. Acute lesions in the posterior and lateral parts of the hypothalamus may be associated with stupor.

46. What is Kleine-Levin syndrome?

Ans. i. It is a periodic somnolence and bulemia.

ii. Episodic disorder characterized by somnolence and over-eating.

iii. Hypothalamus has been implicated.

47. What is the relationship of venous bed to syncope?

Ans. Approximately three-fourths of the systemic blood volume is contained in the venous blood and any interference in venous return may lead to a reduction in cardiac output.

48. What prevents pooling of blood in the lower limb?

Ans. 1. Pressor reflexes that induce constriction of peripheral arterioles and venules.

2. Reflex acceleration of the heart by means of aortic and carotid reflexes.

3. Improvement of venous return to the heart by activity of the muscles of the limb.

49. What is the correlation of orthostatic hypotension with syncope?

Ans. i. Orthostatic hypotension may be the cause of syncope in up to 30% of the elderly.

ii. Polypharmacy with antihypertensives or antidepressant drugs is often a contributor in these patients.

50. What is cardiovascular syncope?

Ans. i. In normal individuals, heart rate between 30 and 180 beats per minute does not reduce cerebral blood flow especially if the person is in the supine position.

ii. a. Digoxin

b. β-adrenoreceptor antagonists

c. Calcium channel blockers and antiarrhythmic drugs may suppress sinoatrial node impulse generation or slow AV nodal conduction.

13 Normal Development and Aging

1. What is the approximate future height of a child (mid-parental height)?

Ans. The approximate future height of a child (mid-parental height) can be simply predicted from the parental heights.
For a boy: Maternal height + 14 cm (5.5 inches) + parental height/2
For a *girl*: Paternal height − 14 cm (5.5 inches) + maternal height/2.

2. What is Moro response?

Ans. It is the infant's reaction to startle and it can be evoked by suddenly withdrawing support of the head and allowing the neck to extend.
This response is present in all newborns and infants up to 4 to 5 months of age and its absence indicates a profound disorder of the motor system.

3. What is tonic neck reflex?

Ans. It consists of extension of the arm and leg on the side to which the head is passively turned and flexion of the opposite limbs. Persistence beyond 6 months represents a malfunction of the nervous system.

4. What is the placing reaction?

Ans. In placing reaction, the foot or hand brought into contact with the edge of the table is lifted automatically and placed on the flat surface. It is present in all newborns.
Its absence or asymmetry under 6 months of age indicates a motor abnormality.

5. What is Landau maneuver?

Ans. The infant if suspended horizontally in the prone position will extend the neck and trunk and will break the trunk extension when the neck is passively flexed. This reaction is present by 6 months. Its delayed appearance in a hypotonic child is indicative of a faulty motor apparatus.

6. What is parachute response?

Ans. If an infant is held prone in the horizontal position and is then dropped towards the bed, an extension of the arm is evoked as if to break the fall. It is elicitable in most 9 months old infants.

7. When does the corticospinal tract get myelinated?

Ans. Corticospinal tract is not fully myelinated until 18 months.

8. What is floppy (hypotonic) infant?

Ans. a. Werdnig Hoffmann's disease
b. Muscular dystrophies and congenital myopathies
c. Maternal myasthenia gravis
d. Polyneuropathies
e. Down's syndrome
f. Prader-Willi syndrome
g. Spinal cord injuries.

9. What is arthrogryposis?

Ans. Hypotonia that arises in utero may be accompanied by congenital fixed contracture of the joints.

10. What are the causes of congenital deafness?

Ans. a. History of familial deaf mutism
b. Congenital rubella
c. Erythroblastosis fetalis
d. Meningitis
e. Chronic bilateral ear infections
f. Administration of ototoxic drugs to the pregnant women or newborn infant.

11. What is idioglossia (congenital word deafness)?

Ans. Word deaf children may chatter incessantly and often adopt a language of their own design which the patient comes to understand. This peculiar type of speech is known as idioglossia.

12. What is stuttering and stammering?

Ans. Essentially they represent a disorder of rhythm. An involuntary repetitive prolongation of speech due to an insuppressible spasm of articulatory muscles.

13. What is the genetics and treatment of attention–deficit hyperactivity disorder?

Ans. i. There is an association between ADHD and a polymorphism of the gene that codes for the same dopamine transporter gene.

ii. *Treatment*:
  • *Methylphenidate*: 5 to 30 mg
  • *Dextramphetamine*: 2.5 to 5 mg three times daily.

14. What is enuresis?

Ans. If a child above 5 years of age wets bed, it is known as nocturnal enuresis.
Causes:
• Spina bifida
• Boy: Obstruction of bladder neck
• Girl: Ectopic ureter entering vagina.

15. Grade mental retardation.

Ans. *Mildly impaired*: IQ 45 to 70.
Severely impaired : IQ below 45.

16. What is gerontology?

Ans. It is a study of aging.

17. What is sarcopenia?

Ans. Many processes contribute to the age-dependent loss of lean muscle mass. This is known as sarcopenia.

14 Inherited Metabolic Diseases of the Nervous System

1. What is diathesis?

Ans. It is a constitutional predisposition.

2. What is the frequency of genetic disorder?

Ans. Of the 10 in every 1000 live births with genetic disorders,
- 7 are dominant
- 2.5 are recessive
- The remainder are sex-linked.

3. What is leukodystrophy? What is poliodystrophy?

Ans. 1. *Leukodystrophy*: (Disorders of cerebral white matter, oligodendrocyte and myelin)
- Early onset of spastic paralysis of the limbs
- With or without ataxia
- Visual impairment with optic atrophy but normal retina

2. *Poliodystrophy (gray matter disease)*:
- Early onset of seizures and myoclonus
- Blindness and retinal changes
- Mental regression.

4. What are the characteristic features of mitochondrial disorders?

Ans. There are two characteristic features:
- Ragged red fibres
- Systemic lactic acidosis

5. What are the metabolic disorders of the neonatal period?

Ans. a. Disorders of amino acid
b. Disorders of ammonia
c. Disorders of organic acid metabolism.
They usually have features to gain weight.

6. What are the hereditary metabolic disorders of infancy?

Ans. a. Leukodystrophies
b. Lysosomal storage disorders.

7. What is Tay-Sach's disease? What is cherry red spot?

Ans. In Tay-Sach's disease, there is
Deficiency of hexosaminidase A and abnormal startle to acoustic stimuli. In *cherry red spot*, degeneration of the macula cells exposes the underlying red vascular choroid.

8. What is infantile Gaucher's disease?

Ans. i. Persistent retroflexion of the neck, strabismus and enlarged spleen.
ii. A deficiency of glucocerebrocidase in leukocytes and hepatocytes is diagnostic.
iii. Increase in serum acid phosphatase and characteristic histiocytes (Gaucher cells).
Classic triad:
• Trismus
• Strabismus
• Opisthotonus.

9. What is infantile Niemann-Pick disease?

Ans. i. Enlargement of liver, spleen, lymph nodes and infiltration of the lungs.
ii. Vacuolated histiocytes (foam cells) in the bone marrow and vacuolated blood lymphocytes.
iii. A deficiency of sphingomyelinase.

10. What is Gm$_1$ gangliosidosis?

Ans. i. Dysmorphic facial features

    ii. Lack of psychomotor development

   iii. Loss of vision, course nystagmus and strabismus, macular cherry red-spot

   iv. A partial or complete deficiency of β-galactosidase

    v. The disease should be suspected in an infant having the facial features of mucopolysaccharidosis and severe early onset neurologic abnormalities.

11. What is Krabbe's disease?

Ans. i. Generalised rigidity

    ii. Opisthotonic curvature of the neck and trunk

   iii. Neuropathy

   iv. Galactocerebrosidase is deficient.

12. What is Farber's disease?

Ans. i. Deficiency of ceramidase

    ii. Periarticular and subcutaneous swellings and progressive arthropathy.

13. What is sudanophilic leukodystrophy and Pelizaus-Merzbacher disease?

Ans. a. Abnormal movements of the eyes

    b. This disease and Cockayne syndromes are the only leukodystrophies in which nystagmus has been an invariable finding.

14. What is Canavan's disease?

Ans. i. Rapid regression of psychomotor function, loss of sight and optic atrophy.

    ii. Attenuation of cerebral and cerebellar white matter in an enlarged brain and relatively normal sized ventricles.

15. What is Alexander disease?

Ans. 1. Failure to thrive, psychomotor retardation, spasticity of the craniospinal musculature and seizures

    2. Progressive macrocephaly

    3. Rosetted fibres.

16. What is cerebrohepatorenal (Zellweger's) disease (peroxisomal disorder)?

Ans. 1. Very long chain fatty acids

2. Dysmorphic alteration of the skull and face

3. Stippled irregular calcification of the patella, greater trochanter are highly characteristic.

17. What is oculocerebrorenal (Lowe) syndrome?

Ans. i. Bilateral cataracts

ii. Renal tubular acidosis and renal failure.

18. What is Menke's disease?

Ans. i. Failure of absorption of copper from GIT

ii. Hair breaks easily and appears twisted (pili torti)

iii. Hypothermia

iv. Metaphyseal spurring and tortuosity and elongation of cerebral and systemic arteries.

19. On what factors does the diagnosis of inherited metabolic disorders of infancy depend on?

Ans. It depends on:

i. Dysmorphic features

ii. Visceromegaly

iii. Purely neurological.

20. What are the features of phenylketonuria?

Ans. 1. Impairment of psychomotor development (mental retardation)

2. Hyperactivity

3. Repetitive digital mannerisms

4. High level of serum phenylalanine and phenylpyruvic acid in the blood, CSF and urine.

21. What are the features of hereditary tyrosinemia (oculocutaneous tyrosinemia)?

Ans. Self mutilation and incoordination of limb movement.

22. What are the features of Hartnup disease?

Ans. 1. Intermittent red scaly rash over the face, neck, hands and legs
2. Emotional lability
3. Episodic cerebellar ataxia
4. *Treatment*: Avoid exposure to sulfonamides and sunlight.

23. What are the features of ataxia-telangiectasia?

Ans. 1. Characterstic telangiectatic lesions on bulbar conjunctiva
2. Decrease in serum immunoglobulins
3. Recurrent pulmonary infections.

24. What are the features of metachromatic leukodystrophy?

Ans. 1. Presence of metachromatic granules in glial cells and macrophage
2. Elevated CSF protein and a marked increase in sulfatide in urine and absence of arylsulfatase.

25. What is the characteristic feature of early childhood Niemann-Pick disease?

Ans. Paralysis of horizontal and vertical gaze.

26. What are the characteristic features of neuronal ceroid lipofuscinosis?

Ans. 1. Widespread myoclonus
2. Retinal degeneration.

27. What are the characteristic features of mucopoly-saccharidosis?

Ans. Neurologic and skeletal abnormalities are present.

28. Discuss Cockayne syndrome.

Ans. a. Stunting of growth
b. Photosensitivity of the skin
c. Retinitis pigmentosis, cataracts, pendular nystagmus
d. Delayed psychomotor development
e. Ataxia of limbs.

29. What are the features of Bassen-Kornzweig acanthocytosis (abetalipoprotinemia)?

Ans. 1. Acanthocytes
2. Reduction in serum of low density lipoproteins
3. Vitamin E is decreased
4. Cerebellar signs are present.

30. Discuss Wilson's disease.

Ans. 1. It is related to copper metabolism.
2. A notable feature is the tendency for motor disorder to be concentrated in the bulbar musculature.
3. Kayser-Fleisher ring (rusty-brown discolouration) They are invariably present once the neurologic signs become manifest.
4. *Treatment*: D-penicillamine 40 mg and liver transplantation.

31. Discuss Hallervorden-Spatz disease.

Ans. 1. It is related to iron metabolism.
2. *Eye of the tiger sign*: T_2 weighted MRI shows areas of decreased signal intensity of the pallidum bilaterally (corresponding to iron deposition) and a central high signal area due to necrosis.
3. *Treatment*: L-dopa.

32. What is Lesch-Nyhan syndrome?

Ans. Essentially it is a:
• Hereditary choreoathetosis
• Self-mutilation
• Hyperurecemia.

33. What is adrenoleukodystrophy?

Ans. i. Excess of very long chain fatty acids
ii. Adrenal glands get affected
Treatment: Adrenal replacement.

34. What are the strokes associated with inherited metabolic disorder?

Ans. • *Homocystinuria*: Treatment 50 to 500 mg of pyridoxine

ii. *Fabry's disease*: Angiokeratoma periumbilically—enzymatic treatment

iii. Sulfite oxidase deficiency

iv. Tangier's disease and familiar hypercholesterolemia.

35. How to suspect adult forms of inherited metabolic disorder?

Ans. The multiplicity of neuronal system involvement is more common in heritable metabolic disease than degenerative disease.

36. Discuss mitochondrial disorders.

Ans. a. Mitochondrial myopathies

b. PEO (progressive external ophthalmoplegia) and kearns-Sayre syndrome

c. Subacute necrotizing encephalopathy (Leigh disease)

d. NARP (neuropathy, ataxia, retinitis, pigmentosis syndrome)

e. Congenital lactic acidosis and recurrent ketoacidemia

f. MERRF: Myoclonic epilepsy with ragged red fibre myopathy

g. MELAS: Mitochondrial, myopathy, encephalopathy, lactic acidosis and stroke like episodes.

37. What are the diagnostic features of mitochondrial disorders?

Ans. 1. Ischaemic forearm test:

a. Measurement of the partial pressure of oxygen in the venous blood from the forearm after exercise (causes relative ischaemia)

b. A paradoxical rise of PO_2 from an average of 27 mmHg

2. Ragged red fibres.

3. Lactic acidosis.

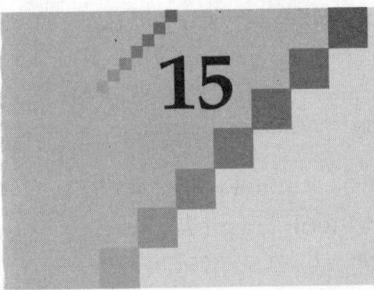

15 Developmental Diseases of the Nervous System

1. What is teratology?

Ans. Teratology is the scientific study of neurosomatic malformations.

2. Why nervous system development is susceptible to disorders?

Ans. Nervous system of all organ systems requires the longest time for its development and maturation during which it is susceptible to disorders.

3. What is hydrencephalus?

Ans. Hydrencephalus is the destruction or failure of the development of parts of the cerebrum.

4. What is porencephaly?

Ans. Porencephaly is the apposition of ventricular and pial surfaces.

5. What is schizencephaly?

Ans. Schizencephaly is the localized failure of evagination.

6. What are the disturbances of neuronal migration?

Ans. Neuroembryologic studies have identified several milestones of:

    i. Neuroblast formation

    ii. Migration

    iii. Cortical organization

iv. Neuronal differentiation

v. Connectivity

During the first trimester of gestation, post-mitotic neurons that will ultimately reside in the cortex area is the ventricular zone adjacent to the ventricle. They then migrate along the scaffold of radial glia to form multilayered cortex.

7. What is holoporencephaly?

Ans. In holoporencephaly emergence of two separate cerebral hemispheres may not occur.

8. What is lissencephaly?

Ans. In lissencephaly, cortical involutions may be absent altogether and there is morphologic evidence of several types of neuroblast deficiency resulting from either generalized or restricted form of neuronal migration. Cortex may fail to become sulcated.

9. What is pachygraphy?

Ans. Pachygraphy is a broad gyral pattern.

10. What is the normal weight of the brain?

Ans. 1000 to 1500 grams.

11. What is encephalocele?

Ans. An eventration of brain tissue and its coverings through an unfused midline defect in the skull is encephalocele.

12. What is Dandy Walker syndrome?

Ans. A failure of the development of the midline portion of the cerebellum is Dandy Walker syndrome.

13. What are the dreaded complications of spinal defects?

Ans. The two dreaded complications of spinal defects are:
 • Meningitis
 • Progressive hydrocephalus from a chiari malformation.

14. What is tethered cord?

Ans. Attachment of (tether) the cord to the sacrum is tethered cord.

15. What is Diastematomyelia?

Ans. When a long spicule or fibrous band protrudes into the spinal canal from the body of the thoracic or upper vertebrae and divides the spinal cord in two halves for a variable vertical extent, it is known as diastematomyelia.

16. What are the types of chiari malformations?

Ans. *Type I*: Cerebellomedullary malformation without meningo-myelocele

Type II: Cerebellomedullary malformation with a meningo-myelocele

Type III: Meningomyelocele with cerebellar herniation

Type IV: Cerebellar hypoplasia.

17. Discuss tuberous sclerosis.

Ans. i. *Due to limited hyperplasia of ectoderm*: Skin, CNS and mesodermal cells

ii. *Clinical triad*:
  - Adenoma sebaceum
  - *Epilepsy*: Flexor spasms—ACTH is the treatment
  - Mental retardation.

18. Discuss neurofibromatosis.

Ans. a. *Neurofibromatosis type I*: Classic or peripheral NF
  - Café-au-lait spots: More than six, size more than 1.5 cm is diagnostic.
  - Molluscum fibrosus
  - Leisch nodules (Hamartomas of the iris)

b. *Neurofibromatosis Type II*: Central or acoustic
  - Bilateral acoustic neuromas.

19. Discuss Sturge-Weber syndrome. (Meningo or encephalofacial angiomatosis with cerebral calcification, encephalotrigeminal syndrome).

Ans. 1. Vascular nevus in the territory of the ophthalmic division of the trigeminal nerve.

    2. Tramline calcification which outlines the convolutions of the paretio-occipital cortex.

    3. Epilepsy.

20. What is Osler-Rendu-Weber disease (hereditary haemorrhagic telengectasia)?

Ans. The basic lesion is probably a defect in the vessel wall and the main complication bleeding is thought to be due to mechanical fragility of the vessel wall.

21. What is von Hippel-Lindau disease?

Ans. This disease has hemangioblastomas:

    i. Cerebellar hemangioblastomas

    ii. Retinal hemangioblastomas.

22. What is Mobius syndrome?

Ans. Bifacial and abducens palsies due to restricted abnormalities of the nervous system.

23. What are the features of cerebral palsy (congenital abnormalities of motor function)?

Ans. 1. Matrix (subependymal) haemorrhage in immature infant (periventricular)

    2. Hypoxic ischaemic encephalopathy (little disease)

    3. Certain developmental motor abnormalities.

24. What is double athetosis?

Ans. Status marmoratus: Whitish strands represent foci of nerve cell loss and gliosis with condensation of bands of traversing myelinated fibres.

25. What is the tetrad in rubella infections?

Ans. i. Cataract

    ii. Deafness

    iii. Congenital heart disease

    iv. Mental retardation.

26. What is the Hutchinson's triad in congenital neurosyphilis?

Ans. 1. Dental deformities
   2. Interstitial keratitis
   3. Bilateral deafness.

27. What are the epilepsies of infancy and childhood?

Ans. a. Benign neonatal convulsions
   b. Benign myoclonic epilepsy of infancy
   c. Febrile seizures (both genetic and acquired)
   d. Infantile spasms of the west
   e. Absence seizures
   f. Lennox-Gestaut syndrome
   g. Rolandic and occipital paraxosms and other benign focal epilepsies
   i. Juvenile myoclonic epilepsy.

28. What is hereditary mental retardation?

Ans. 1. Fragile X-syndrome (seen in boys)
   2. Rett syndrome (seen in girls): Hand wringing is characteristic feature.
   3. William syndrome: Supravalvular aortic stenosis and musical interest.

29. What is autism (Kanner-Asperger syndrome)?

Ans. A social, lacking in communicative skills both verbal and nonverbal and committed to repetitive ritualistic behaviours.

16 Acquired Metabolic Disorders and Related Disorders of the Nervous System

1. What is the formula for serum osmolality?

Ans. Serum osmolality = 2[Na + K] + Glucose/18 + BUN/3.

2. What is autoregulation?

Ans. Autoregulation is compensatory dilatation of resistance vessels in response to a reduction in cerebral perfusion which maintains blood flow at a constant rate.

3. What are the nervous structures which are vulnerable to hypoxia?

Ans. a. With anoxia neurons in portions of the hippocampus and the deep fibres of the cerebellum are particularly vulnerable.

b. The nucleus structures of the brain stem and spinal cord are relatively resistant to anoxia and hypotension and stop functioning only after the cortex has been badly damaged.

4. When anoxic encephalopathy does not cause permanent damage?

Ans. Degree of hypoxia that at no time abolish consciousness rarely if ever causes permanent damage to the nervous system.

5. What is no-flow phenomenon or irreversibility?

Ans. One of the reasons for the irreversibility of the lesions may be swelling of the endothelium and blockage of the circulation into the ischaemic cerebral arteries, the so-called no-flow phenomenon.

6. What prolongs the tolerability period of brain to hypoxia?

Ans. Subnormal body temperature as might occur when the body is immersed in the ice-cold water, greatly prolongs the tolerability period of brain to hypoxia.

7. What are the early changes of hypoxic encephalopathy?

Ans. The most common early changes in cases of severe injury is a loss of distinction between the cerebral gray matter and white matter.

8. What are watershed infarctions?

Ans. With less severe and predominantly hypotensive-ischaemic cortex such as cardiac arrest, watershed infarctions become evident in the border zones between the anterior, middle and posterior cerebral arteries.

Types:

a. *Between middle and posterior cerebral arteries*: Visual agnosias including Balint's syndrome and cortical blindness represents infarction of the watershed between middle and posterior cerebral arteries.

b. *Between middle and anterior cerebral arteries*: Proximal arm and shoulder weakness, sometimes accompanied by hip weakness (referred to as a man in the Barrel syndrome) reflects infarction in the territory between middle and anterior cerebral arteries. The patients are able to walk, but their arms dangle and their hips may be weak.

9. What does hypercapnia (increased CO_2) cause?

Ans. • Papilledema
• Asterixes.

10. Correlate blood sugar level with brain state. What is incretin effect?

Ans. a. The glucose reserve (1 to 2 gm) will sustain cerebral activity for only about 30 minutes once the blood glucose is no longer available.
• *Below 30 mg*: Confusion
• *Below 10 mg*: Coma (medullary phase)

b. *Incretin effect*: It is known that the insulin response to oral glucose is greater than the response to intravenous glucose. This is known as the incretin effect and is due to release of two peptide hormones, glucose-dependent insulinotropic peptide (GIP) and glucagon-like peptide-1 (GLP-1) from the L cells in the intestine.

11. What causes brain edema during the treatment of hyperglycemia?

Ans. The brain edema in this condition is probably due to the reversal of the osmolality gradient from blood to brain which occurs with rapid correction of hyperglycemia.

12. What is Reye's syndrome?

Ans. a. It is due to aspirin intake in children.

b. *Treatment*: Anti-edema measures.

13. Correlate AEDS with uremic encephalopathy.

Ans. Convulsions which occur in about one-third of cases, often preterminally may respond to relatively low plasma concentration of anti-convulsants – the reason being that serum albumin is depressed in uremia, increasing the unbound therapeutically active portion of the drug.

14. Discuss hepatic encephalopathy.

Ans. 1. Asterixis (sterixis indicates a fixed position): Characteristic intermittency of sustained muscle contraction
2. EEG: Triphasic waves in delta range
3. Blood ammonia is more than 200 mg per dl
4. Neuropathologically, there is an increase in the number and size of the protoplasmic astrocytes in the deep layers of the cerebral cortex.
5. False neurotransmitters: Phenols/short chain fatty acids octapamine, mercaptans and manganese
6. Pathogenesis:
   • Ammonia
   • GABA nergic benzodiazepine hypothesis
     Treatment: Flumazenil

7. *Treatment*:
- Restriction of dietary proteins
- Oral neomycin
- Enema
- Oral lactulose that reduces bacterial activity.

15. What is central pontine myelinosis?

Ans. a. Usually seen in alcoholics.
   b. Mostly due to rapid correction or over correction of hyponatremia.
   c. Hyponatremia to be corrected by no more than 10 mEq/L in the initial 24 hours and by no more than 21 mEq/L in initial 48 hours.

16. What are the acquired metabolic disorders presenting as psychosis and dementia?

Ans. a. Cushing's disease and corticosteroid psychosis
   b. Thyroid encephalopathies
   c. Pancreatic encephalopathy.

17. What is Wernicke's disease?

Ans. Nystagmus, abducens and conjugate gaze palsy, ataxia of gait and mental confusion due to thiamine deficiency is known as Wernicke's disease.

18. What is Korsakoff amnesic state?

Ans. *Korsakoff psychosis*: Retentive memory is impaired.

19. What is the triad of Wernicke's disease?

Ans. Triad of Wernicke's disease:
- Ophthalmoplegia
- Ataxia
- Disturbance of mentation and confusion.

20. What is Marchiafava-Bignami disease?

Ans. It is primary degeneration of the corpus callosum:
- Due to alcohol
- Front lobe signs are present.

21. Discuss delerium tremens.

Ans. a. Due to rapid decline of alcohol levels

b. 24% develop, 5% fatality

c. They die in a state of hyperthermia

d. Precipitates seizure because of:

 • Reduced magnesium levels

 • Increased arterial pH

e. Always give vitamin B_1 and then glucose

f. Chlordiazepoxide and diazepam are used in controlling withdrawal symptoms.

22. How does alcohol produce hypoglycemia?

Ans. Alcohol produces transient hypoglycemia within 24 hours secondary to acute action of alcohol on gluconeogenesis.

23. Discuss alcohol metabolism in terms of glucose and fat.

Ans. • Alcohol impairs gluconeogenesis in the liver with a resultant fall in the amount of glucose produced from glycogen.

 • Lactate production increases and there is a decreased oxidation of fatty acids with an increase in fat accumulation in liver cells.

24. What are the beneficial effects of moderate alcohol consumption?

Ans. A minimum of one to two drinks per day may decrease the risk of cardiovascular death perhaps through an increase in high density lipoproteins (HDL) cholesterol or changes in clotting mechanism.

25. What are the blood tests for alcoholism?

Ans. • Increase in gamma glutamyl transferase (GGT) levels

 • Carbohydrate deficient transferrrin (CDT) levels.

26. What is the treatment of alcohol withdrawal?

Ans. • Most withdrawal symptoms are caused by the rapid removal of a CNS depressant.

- Patients can be weaned by benzodiazepines and gradually decreasing the levels over 3 to 5 days (25 to 50 mg of chlordiazepoxide every 4 to 6 hours on first day).

27. What is the treatment of alcohol addiction?

Ans. Disulfiram interferes with the metabolism of alcohol so that a patient who takes both alcohol and disulfiram accumulate an inordinate amount of acetaldehyde in the tissues resulting in a nause, vomiting and hypotension.

28. What is pathoclisis?

Ans. Each system of neurons has its own vulnerabilities to particular drugs and toxic agents.

29. What is the effect and treatment of opioid overdose?

Ans. It causes respiratory depression.
Treatment: Naloxone.

30. What is the treatment of opioid abstinence syndrome?

Ans. 1 mg of methadone for 3 mg of morphine.

31. Correlate barbiturate with EEG changes.

Ans. Isoelectric EEG can occur with barbiturate overdose and should not be equated with brain death.

32. Describe neuroleptic malignant syndrome.

Ans. i. Most dreaded complication of phenothiazine and haloperidol use.

ii. The syndrome consists of rigidity, stupor, unstable blood pressure, variable hyperthermia, disphoresis and other signs of autonomic dysfunction, high serum creatinine (up to 60,000) and renal failure due to myo-globinuria.

iii. *Treatment*: Bromocriptine 5 mg tid (up to 20 mgs tid) will terminate the condition in few hours.

33. Who are body packers and body stuffers?

Ans. *Body packers (also known as mules)*: They are individuals who attempt to smuggle drugs across national borders or into prisons by ingesting multiple small packets that are swallowed for later retrieval from vomit or faeces or are inserted into the vagina or rectum.

Body stuffers: In contrast, body stuffers are individuals who ingest drugs to avoid detection or arrest by the police.

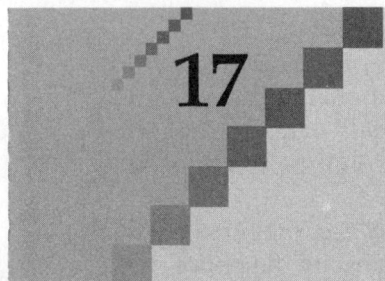

17 Infections of the Nervous System

1. What are Kerning's and Brudzinski's signs?

Ans. *Kerning's sign*: With the hip joint flexed, extension of the knee causes spasm of the hamstring muscles.
Brudzinski's sign: Passive flexion of the neck causes flexion of the thigh and knees.

2. What is the etiology of meningitis according to age?

Ans. 1. *Adults*:
- *Streptococcus pneumoniae*
- *Neisseria meningitis*
- *Hemophilus influenzae*
- *Listeria monocytogenes*

2. *Neonate*:
- *Escherchia coli*
- Group B Streptococcus

3. *Infant and child*:
- *Hemophilus infuenzae*

4. *Neurosurgical circumstances*:
- Staphylococci
- *Listeria monocytogenes.*

3. What are the frequencies of organisms responsible for community acquired bacterial meningitis?

Ans. a. *Streptococcus pneumoniae* (50%)
b. *N. meningitis* (25%)
c. Group B Streptococcus (15%)

d. *Listeria monocytogenes* (10%)

e. *H. influenzae* (less than 10%)

f. *Entreic gram*-negative bacilli

g. *Staphylococcus aureus* (following invasive neurosurgical procedures).

4. How does meningococcus invade?

Ans. Meningococcus invades through nasopharynx.

5. How does *Streptococcus pnuemoniae* and *H. influenzae* invade?

Ans. They invade through otitis media.

6. What are the various modes of spread of pyogenic infections?

Ans. Reach the intracranial structures by two pathways:

- Haematogenous spread
- Extension from cranial structures.

7. What is Hubener's arteritis?

Ans. The striking feature of subintimal fibrosis is present in nearly all types of subacute and chronic infections of the meninges, but most notably of tuberculosis and syphilitic meningitis.

8. What are the pathologic–clinical correlations in acute, subacute and chronic meningial reactions?

Ans. I. **In acute meningial infections:**

     a. *Pure pia–arachnoiditis*: Forward flexion of the neck (Brudzinski's sign) and extension of legs (Kerning's sign) involve maneuvers that oppose the protective flexor reflexes

     b. Subpial encephalopathy

     c. Inflammatory or vascular involvement of cranial nerve roots

     d. Thrombosis of meningial veins

     e. Ependymitis, choroid plexitis

     f. Cerebellar or cerebral hemisphere herniation

II. **Subacute and chronic form of meningitis:**
   a. Tension hydrocephalus
   b. Subdural effusion
   c. Extensive venous or arterial infarction
III. **Late effects or sequelae:**
   a. Meningial fibrosis around optic nerve or around spinal cord or roots
   b. Chronic meningoencephalitis with hydrocephalus
   c. Resistant hydrocephalus in the child.

9. What is the significance of neck stiffness?

Ans. i. Present only or predominantly on forward flexion
   ii. Initial few degrees are specific
   iii. Later few degrees are sensitive.

10. What are the signs of raised ICP?

Ans. i. CSF pressure is usually more than 180 mm of water.
   ii. *Cushing reflex*:
   • Bradycardia
   • Hypertension
   • Irregular respiration.

11. Discuss CSF glucose status.

Ans. i. It takes from 30 minutes to several hours for CSF glucose concentration to reach equilibrium with blood glucose concentration.
   ii. A CSF/serum glucose ratio of less than 0.4 is highly suggestive of bacterial meningitis.

12. What is a specific test of CSF diagnosis of bacterial meningitis?

Ans. The latex agglutination (LA test) is specific.

13. Correlate MRI with meningitis.

Ans. i. In patients with bacterial meningitis diffuse, meningial enhancement is often seen after the administration of gadolinium.

ii. Meningial enhancement is not diagnostic of meningitis but occurs in any CNS disease associated with increased blood–brain barrier permeability.

14. Discuss CSF profile of meningitis.

Ans. i. *Viral CNS infections*: Lymphocytic pleocytosis with normal glucose contents

ii. *Fungal/TB infections*: Lymphocytic pleocytosis with low glucose

iii. *Bacterial meningitis*: PMN pleocytosis with hypoglycorrhachia

iv. Lactic acid is elevated in both bacterial and fungal meningitis but is normal in viral meningitis.

15. What is the empirical anti-microbial therapy?

Ans. a. Community acquired bacterial meningitis:
- *S. pneumoniae, N. meningitis*: Ceftriaxone
- *L. monocytogenes*: Ampicillin

b. Hospital acquired meningitis:
- *Staphylococci seen in neurosurgical conditions*: Neurosurgical treatment
- *Pseudomonas*: Vancomycin, ceftazidime.

16. Discuss the role of steroids in meningitis.

Ans. i. Dexamethasone intravenously 10 mg to be administered 15 to 20 minutes before the first dose of an anti-microbial agent and the same dose repeated every 6 hours for 4 days.

ii. It is unlikely to be of significant benefit if started more than 6 hours after anti-microbial therapy has been initiated.

iii. Dexamethasone exerts its beneficial effect by
a. Inhibiting the synthesis of IL-1 and TNF at the level of mRNA
b. Decreasing CSF outflow resistance
c. Stabilizing the blood–brain barrier

iv. The benefits were most striking with pneumococcal meningitis.

v. In children predominantly with meningitis due to *H. influenzae* and *S. pneumoniae,* steroids are efficacious in decreasing meningeal inflammation and neurological sequelae such as the incidence of sensory—neural hearing loss.

17. Discuss meningococcal meningitis.

Ans. i. Evolution is extremely rapid.

ii. Petechial rash is present in 50%.

iii. Circulatory shock may be present.

iv. A seven-day course of intravenous antibiotic therapy is adequate for uncomplicated meningococcal meningitis.

v. *Chemoprophylaxis (close contacts)*: Rifampicin 600 mg every 12 hours for 2 days in adults and 10 mg/kg every 12 hours for two days in children for more than one year.

vi. Rifampicin is not recommended for pregnant women.

18. Discuss pneumococcal meningitis.

Ans. i. Cranial nerve abnormalities are present

ii. Focal cerebral signs

iii. Seen in splenectomized patients

iv. A two-week course of intravenous anti-microbial therapy is recommended for pneumococcal meningitis.

19. What is common in *H. influenzae* meningitis?

Ans. Seizures are common in *H. influenzae* meningitis.

20. What are the causes of focal and generalized seizures?

Ans. *Focal seizures*:
- Focal arterial ischaemia
- Cortical vein thrombosis
- Edema

Generalized seizures:
- Hyponatremia
- Cerebral anoxia.

21. Discuss neonatal meningitis.

Ans. i. Occurs at or near the time of birth.

ii. The most significant factor in the pathogenesis of the meningitis is maternal infection (usually urinary tract infection or peuperal fever of unknown cause.

iii. *Causative organisms*: *E. coli*, group B Streptococcus.

22. What are the causes of recurrent bacterial meningitis?

Ans. a. CSF rhinorrhea

b. Ventricular-peritoneal shunt infection.

23. Differentiate between CSF rhinorrhea and watery nasal discharge.

Ans. In CSF rhinorrhea, the amount of glucose approximates that obtained by lumbar puncture.

24. What is the treatment of *L. monocytogenes* meningitis?

Ans. *L. monocytogenes* meningitis is treated with ampicillin for at least three weeks.

25. What is the treatment of staphylococcal meningitis?

Ans. Vancomycin is the drug of choice for methicillin-resistant staphylococci.

26. What is the treatment of gram-negative bacillary meningitis?

Ans. i. A three-week course of IV antibiotics (ceftriaxone or ceftazidime)

ii. *P. aeruginosa* should be treated with ceftazidime.

27. Discuss the treatment of meningitis.

Ans. i. Ampicillin for listeria monocytogenes.

ii. Ceftazidime or cefpime (fourth-generation cephalosporin) for *P. aeruginosa*.

iii. Most cases of bacterial meningitis should be treated for a period of 10 to 14 days except when there is a persistent parameningeal focus of infection (otitic or sinus origin).

iv. *Corticosteroids*:

Children: Should include dexamethasone 0.15 mg per kg four times daily for 4 days especially *H. influenzae* meningitis.

Adults:

a. Dexamethasone 10 mg is given just before the first dose of antibiotics and every six hours for four days.

b. Especially for pneumococcal infections, overwhelming infection: very high CSF pressure or signs of herniation, high CSF bacterial count with minimal pleocytosis and signs of acute adrenal insufficiency, i.e. water house-Fredrichson's syndrome).

v. *Anti-convulsants*:

a. If seizure has occurred

b. Cortical vein occlusion

vi. *Prophylaxis*:

a. Single dose of ciprofloxacin

b. Oral dose of rifampicin 600 mg every 12 hours in adults and 10 mg per kg every 12 hours in children for two days.

28. What is the prognosis in meningitis?

Ans. *Mortality*:

- *H. influenzae, N. meningitis*, group B Streptococcus: 5%
- *L. monocytogenes*: 15%
- *S. pneumoniae*: 20%
- Cranial nerve palsies other than deafness tends to disappear after a few weeks or months. Deafness is due to either cochlear destruction or aminoglycoside antibiotics.

29. Discuss brain abscess.

Ans. a. 40% of all brain abscesses are related to diseases of paranasal sinuses, middle ear and mastoid cells.

b. Temporal lobe gets frequently affected followed by cerebellum.

c. About 1/3rd (33%) of all brain abscesses are metastatic, i.e. haematogenous metastatic abscesses are frequently multiple.

d. The distinction between a brain abscess and tumour may be facilitated with diffusion weighted imaging (DWI) sequences in which brain abscess typically shows increased signal and low apparent diffusion coefficient.

30. What are mycotic aneurysms?

Ans. The inflamed artery may form an aneurysm (mycotic aneurysm) that later gives rise to parenchymal or sub-arachnoid haemorrhage.

31. What is the association of cerebral abscess with children?

Ans. In children, more than 60% of cerebral abscesses are associated with congenital heart disease (TOF being the commonest).

32. Discuss the etiology of cerebral abscess.

Ans. The most common organisms causing the brain abscesses are: Streptococcus, Staphylococci.
- Staphylococcal abscesses are due to accidental or surgical trauma.
- Anaerobic streptococci are due to metastasis from lungs and paranasal sinuses.
- Enteric organisms are associated with otitic infections.

33. Discuss TB meningitis.

Ans. i. In 2/3rd of patients with TBM, there is evidence of active tuberculosis elsewhere.

ii. Except for the emergence of drug-resistant organisms, the HIV infection does not appear to change the clinical manifestations or the outcome of TBM.

iii. *Treatment*: INH, ethionamide and pyrazinamide penetrate the blood–brain barrier better than other drugs.

iv. Corticosteroids are used along with ATT in:
   a. Raised ICT
   b. Subarachnoid block (hydrocephalus) for about four weeks.

v. Mortality is 10%.

34. Discuss neurosyphilis.

Ans. a. *Principal types*:
- Asymptomatic neurosyphilis
- Meningial syphilis
- Meningovascular syphilis:
  - Most common form of neurosyphilis
  - Hubner's arteritis
- Paretic neurosyphilis (general paresis)
- Tabetic neurosyphilis (tabes dorsalis):
  - Ataxia is the most prominent feature
  - Charcot's joints (destruction of the articular surfaces) due to repeated injury to an anesthetic joint
  - Visceral crisis: Intestinal crisis with colic and diarrhea
- Syphilitic optic atrophy
- Spinal syphilis
  - Syphilitic meningomyelitis (sometimes called Erb's spastic paraplegia because of the predominance of bilateral corticospinal tract signs
  - Spinal meningovascular syphilis

b. *Treatment of neurosyphilis*:
  a. Penicillin G 40 lakhs fourth hourly for 14 days
  b. Erythromycin/tetracycline 0.5 gram every 6 hours for 20 to 30 days.

35. Discuss cryptococcal meningitis.

Ans. *Diagnosis*: Indian ink preparation
Treatment:
- Intravenous amphotericin 0.5 to 0.7 mg/kg/day. Stop if BUN reaches 40 mg/day.
- Flucytosine 150 mg/kg/day: Causes neutropenia
  - Both can be combined so as to reduce the dose of amphotericin from 0.3 to 0.5 mg/kg/day. Treatment is given for 6 weeks.
- Fluconazole: 400 mg per day.
- The most common complication of fungal meningitis is hydrocephalus.

36. What is Lyme disease?

Ans. i. Caused by B. burgdorferri

ii. *Treatment*: Doxycycline 100 mg bd

iii. Causes facial palsy and meningoradiculitis of cauda equina (Bannwarth syndrome).

37. How does fungal infections of the CNS present?

Ans. i. Subacute meningeal infections

ii. Multi-focal encephalitic disorders.

38. What are opportunistic infections?

Ans. i. Infections related to the impairment of the body's protective mechanisms.

ii. They include fungal infections and also due to certain bacteria, protozoa, viruses.

39. Discuss candidiasis (moniliasis).

Ans. a. Most frequent type of opportunistic fungal infection.

b. Present in severe burns and total parenteral nutrition.

c. *Treatment*: IV amphotericin.

40. Discuss aspergillosis.

Ans. i. Aspergillosis does not present as meningitis but hyphal invasion of cerebral vessels may occur with thrombosis, necrosis and haemorrhage.

ii. Preceded by a pulmonary infection that is unresponsive to antibiotics.

iii. *Treatment*: Amphotericin, itracanazole 200 mg bd.

41. Discuss mucormycosis.

Ans. i. Seen as a complication in patients with diabetic acidosis.

ii. Cerebral infection begins in nasal turbinates.

42. What is the treatment of actinomycosis?

Ans. Penicillin is the treatment of choice for actinomycosis.

43. Discuss toxoplasmosis.

Ans. a. *Seen in immunosuppressive conditions*: AIDS

b. Chorioretinitis, hydrocephalus, cerebral calcifications, psychomotor retardation

c. *Treatment*: Oral sulfadizine, pyrithimine, leucorine.

44. What is the treatment of amoebic meningoencephalitis?

Ans. a. Caused by balamuthia

b. *Treatment*: IV amphotericin B.

45. What is the treatment of trichinosis?

Ans. Thiabendazole, prednisone.

46. Discuss schistosomiasis.

Ans. a. *S. japonicum*: Causes cerebral hemiplegia

b. *S. mansoni*: Affects spinal cord

Treatment: Praziquantel 20 mg/kg tid.

47. Discuss cerebral malaria.

Ans. i. Complicates 2% of cases of falciparium malaria.

ii. Neurological symptoms (headache, coma, seizures, cerebral edema) appear on 2nd or 3rd weeks of infection.

iii. Once coma and convulsions supervene, 20 to 30 percent of patients do not survive.

iv. Dexamathasone at the onset of cerebral symptoms may be life saving.

48. Discuss neurocysticercosis.

Ans. i. Multiple calicified lesions

ii. Before the cyst degenerates and eventually calcifies, CT scanning and MRI may actually visualize the scolex

iii. Commonest neurological presentation: Seizures

iv. Racemose form of the illness

In the most malignant form of the disease, the cysticerci are located in the basal subarachnoid space where they induce an intense inflammatory reaction leading to hydrocephalus, vasculitis, stroke as well as cranial nerve palsies.

Treatment: Praziquantel 50 mg/kg for 15 to 30 days.
Albendazole 5 mg/kg tid for 15 to 30 days.

Corticosteriods:

i. May be useful if a large single lesion is causing symptoms by mass effect.

ii. Anti-epileptic therapy can be stopped once the follow-up CT scan shows resolution of the lesion.

49. What are neurotropic viruses?

Ans. Exhibiting an affinity for certain types of neurons.

Examples:

- Polio virus and motor neurons
- VZV and peripheral sensory neurons
- Rabies virus and brain stem neurons.

50. What are neurohistopathic viruses?

Ans. Involves all elements of the nervous system.

Examples:

- Herpes simplex and medial part of temporal lobe destroying neurons/vessels
- *HIV*: Induces multiple foci of tissue necrosis throughout cerebrum.

51. Discuss various pathways of infection.

Ans. i. Breaks blood–brain barrier (BBB)

ii. Retrograde axoplasmic transport system (HSV, VZV, rabies virus)

iii. HSV may spread to the CNS involving olfactory neurons in the nasal mucosa.

52. What are the causes of chronic and recurrent meningitis?

Ans. i. Vogt-Koyanagi-Harada syndrome:

- Irodocyclitis
- Depigmentation
- Deafness
- Benign and unknown pathology

ii. HSV-I and HSV-II infection (mollaret meningitis)

      iii. Allergic and hypersensitivity meningitis

      iv. Behçets disease.

53. What is the causative organism for the syndrome of acute encephalitis?

Ans. HSV is by far the commonest sporadic cause of encephalitis and has no seasonal or geographical predilection.

54. Discuss HSV encephalitis.

Ans.   i. Commonest and gravest form of acute encephalitis

      ii. Two routes of entry

        a. Through nose

        b. Through trigeminal nerve fibres.

      iii. *EEG*: Lateralized periodic high voltage sharp waves in the temporal region and slow wave high voltage sharp waves in the temporal region and slow wave complexes at regular two to three per second intervals.

      iv. *Treatment*: Acyclovir is given intravenously in a dosage of 30 mg/kg/day and continued for 10 to 14 days.

55. Discuss rabies.

Ans.   i. Incubation period 20 to 60 days

      ii. Hydrophobia due to involvement of tegmental medullary cortex

      iii. *Furious rabies*: Salivation and hydrophobia

          Dumb (paralytic) rabies: Spinal cord gets affected

      iv. *Pathology*: Negri bodies, babes nodules

      v. *Postexposure prophylaxis*: HRIG (human rabies immuno-globulin) 20 u/kg body weight.

          Vaccination: HDCV (human diploid cell vaccine) 5 days on 0, 3, 7, 14, 28.

56. What are the syndromes of herpes zoster?

Ans. a. VZV

        i. Follows a primary infection with chickenpox

        ii. Primarily localized in trigeminal and thoracic ganglion cells ($T_5 - T_{10}$)

iii. *Vesicles*: Appear within 72 to 96 hours
Dries in 5 to 10 days

b. Ophthalmic herpes (V_1)

c. Ramsay Hunt syndrome (geniculate herpes)
Herpes of the geniculate ganglion of 7th nerve consists of a facial palsy in combination with a herpetic eruption of the external auditory meatus sometimes with tinnitus, vertigo and deafness.
Treatment: Oral acyclovir 800 mg 5 times a day for 7 days
For disseminated: IV acyclovir for 10 days
For post-herpetic neuralgia: (5 to 10%) capsacin ointment/amytryptilline/narcotic.

57. What are the neurologic disorders that are induced by retrovirus and opportunistic infections?

Ans. *Retrovirus*: RNA
Lentevirus: AIDS
Oncornavirus:
a. Chronic T-cell leukemia
b. TSP (HIV-2).

58. Discuss SSPE (subacute sclerosing pan encephalitis).

Ans. i. Measles infection before 2 years followed by a 6–8 year asymptomatic period
ii. *EEG*: Periods (every 5 to 8 seconds) bursts of 2–3 per second high voltage followed by a relatively flat pattern
iii. *Treatment*: Inosiplex.

59. What is progressive multifocal leukoencephalopathy (PML)?

Ans. i. PML is a progressive disorder characterized pathologically by multi-focal areas of demylination of varying size distributed throughout CNS.
ii. Clinical features
a. Visual defects (45 %)
b. Mental impairment (38%)
c. Motor weakness (75%).

iii. Patients have an underlying immunosuppressive disorder. More than 60 % of usually diagnosed PML cases occur in patients with AIDS.

iv. No effective therapy.

60. What are prion diseases?

Ans. They are both

a. Genetic

b. Infectious.

61. Discuss Creutzfeldt-Jacob disease.

Ans. i. Dementia

ii. Stimulus sensitive myoclonus

iii. *EEG changes*: High voltage (1 to 2 Hz) and sharp wave complexes on an increasingly slow and low voltage background.

18

Multiple Sclerosis

1. What is multiple sclerosis? What are the classic features of multiple sclerosis?

Ans. It is a chronic condition characterized clinically by episodes of focal disorders of the optic nerves, spinal cord and brain, which remit to a varying extent and recur over a period of many years.

The classical features of multiple sclerosis are:

   i. Motor weakness

  ii. Paraparesis

 iii. Loss of sight

 iv. Diplopia

   v. Nystagmus

 vi. Dysarthria

vii. Intention tremor

viii. Ataxia

 ix. Impairment of deep sensation

   x. Bladder dysfunction.

2. What is the triad of multiple sclerosis?

Ans. i. Inflammation

  ii. Demyelination

 iii. Gliosis (scarring).

3. What is the pathology of multiple sclerosis?

Ans. i. Plaque

  ii. Periventricular localization is characteristic.

4. What is the pathogenesis of multiple sclerosis?

Ans. *Molecular mimicry*: A shared antigen between the virus and CNS myelin, the oligodendrocyte or cerebral vessels.

5. What is Uthoff's phenomenon?

Ans. A classic feature of multiple sclerosis is the temporary induction by heat or exercise of symptoms such as unilateral visual blurring or tingling and weakness of a limb.

6. What peculiarity may be seen with the clinical features of multiple sclerosis?

Ans. The patient with multiple sclerosis (MS) presents with symptoms in one leg but with signs in both.

7. What is Lhermitte's sign?

Ans. i. Flexion of the neck may produce a tingling, electric like sensation radiating down the shoulder and back.

ii. It is attributable to an increased sensitivity of demyelinated axons to the stretch or pressure on the spinal cord induced by neck flexion.

8. What is dyschromatopsia?

Ans. i. Dyschromatopsia takes a form of disorder of colour appreciation.

ii. One half or more of adult patients who present with optic neuritis will eventually develop the signs of multiple sclerosis.

9. What is Charcot's triad?

Ans. i. Nystagmus

ii. Scanning speech

iii. Intention tremor.

10. What are the diseases causing INO?

Ans. Unilateral and internuclear ophthalmoplegia may be seen in pontine infarcts but the presence of bilateral internuclear ophthalmoplegia in a young adult is virtually diagnostic of multiple sclerosis.

11. Correlate facial hyperesthesia with MS.

Ans. The occurrence of transient facial hyperesthesia or anesthesia of trigeminal neuralgia in a young adult should always support the diagnosis of MS implicating the intra medullary fibers of the fifth nerve.

12. What are the CSF findings of multiple sclerosis?

Ans. CSF abnormalities found in MS include a mononuclear cell pleocytosis and an increased level of intramedullary synthesized IgG.

13. What is the MRI finding of MS?

Ans. *Dawson's fingers*: Lesions are frequently oriented perpendicular to the ventricular surface corresponding to the pathologic pattern of perivenous demyelination.

14. What are the two phases of multiple sclerosis?

Ans. i. *Inflammation*: Leads to attacks
ii. *Neurodegeneration*: Leads to progression.

15. What is the disease modifying therapy for relapsing form?

Ans. IF-β 1 α (avonex).

16. What is the treatment of acute attacks of multiple sclerosis?

Ans. i. IV methyl prednisolone 500 to 1000 mg per day for 3 to 5 days followed by oral prednisolone beginning at a dose of 60 to 80 mg per day and gradually tapered over 2 weeks.
ii. Plasma exchange.

19

Craniocerebral Trauma

1. What is the significance of trauma?

Ans. In persons under 45 years of age, trauma is the leading cause of death and more than 50% are due to head injuries.

2. What is the role of neurosurgery in trauma?

Ans. Fewer than 20% ever require neurosurgical intervention of any kind.

3. What is battle sign?

Ans. If the fracture extends more posteriorly, damaging the sigmoid sinus, the tissue behind the ear and the mastoid process becomes boggy and discoloured.

4. What is the frequent sequelae of head injury?

Ans. Anosmia.

5. Can trauma produce diabetes insipidus?

Ans. Yes, a fracture in or near the sella may tear the stalk of the pituitary gland resulting in DI.

6. What are the common manifestations of trauma?

Ans. i. Trochlear nerve injury
ii. Carotido-cavernous fistula.

7. What are concussion, contusion and diffuse axonal injury?

Ans. i. *Concussion*: It implies a violent shaking or jarring of the brain and a resulting transient functional impairment.

The shearing stresses are maximal at the point where cerebral hemispheres rotate on the relatively fixed brain stem (i.e. at the midbrain-subthalamic level) which results in concussion.

Anterograde amnesia: The duration of anterograde amnesia is the most reliable index of the severity of the concussion injury.

ii. **Contusion:** Contusion on the other hand, implies bruising of cerebral tissue.

iii. *Diffuse axonal injury*: Nerve fibres are stretched rather than torn.

8. What are the coup and contrecoup lesions?

Ans. *Coup lesion*: Contusion of the surface of the brain beneath the point of impact.

Contrecoup lesion: More extensive laciration and contusion on the side opposite to the site of impact.

9. What are the common sites of cerebral contusion?

Ans. Common sites of cerebral contusion are:
- Frontal lobe
- Temporal lobe.

10. What is the Glasgow Coma Scale in terms of prognosis for head injury?

Ans. *GCS*:
- More than 12: Mild injury
- 8–12: Moderate injury
- Less than 7: Severe injury.

11. What are the MRI signal changes of haematoma?

Ans. T_2
- Initially hypointense due to oxyhaemoglobin
- Subsequent weeks hyperintense due to methemoglobin
- Later again hypointense.

12. What is the role of corticosteroids in haematoma?

Ans. Although no longer a common practice, the administration of corticosteroids is an alternative to surgical removal of subacute and chronic subdural haematoma in patients with mass symptoms or with some contraindications to surgery.

13. Discuss post-traumatic epilepsy.

Ans. Epilepsy is the most common delayed sequelae of cranio-cerebral trauma.

Seen in 5% of patients with closed head injuries and 50% who had sustained a compound skull fracture.

14. What is the medical treatment of craniocerebral trauma?

Ans. i. Normal saline is the ideal fluid.

ii. Bromocriptine with morphine is very effective in patients with autonomic dysfunction syndrome in traumatic coma.

15. What anti-hypertensive should not be used in post-traumatic hypertension (BP 180/95)?

Ans. i. Calcium channel blockers should not be used because they cause subdural vasodilatation, increased cerebral blood volume and elevated ICP.

ii. ACEI, β-blockers and diuretics can be used.

20

Intracranial Neoplasms

1. What are the common brain tumours?

Ans. i. Glial tumours account for 50 to 60% of primary brain tumours

ii. Meningiomas for 25%

iii. Schwannomas for 10%

iv. Metastasis.

2. What are the clinical features of tumour?

Ans. The clinical features are:

1. A headache that worsens rather than ablates with recumbency is suggestive of a mass lesion.

2. Projectile vomiting (vomiting without preceeding nausea)

3. A first seizure during adulthood is always suggestive of a brain tumour.

4. *Clinical sign*: Papilledema: The elevation of the ICP and perioptic pressure impairs axonal transport in the optic nerve and the venous drainage form the optic nerve head and retina manifesting itself as papilledema.

   a. *Primary brain tumour*:

      • Subacute progression of a focal neurologic deficit

      • Seizures

      • Non-focal neurological disorders such as headache, dementia, personality change, gait disorders

   b. *Metastatic tumour*: Malaise, weight loss, anemia.

3. What are false localizing signs?

Ans. Once pressure is raised in a particular compartment of the cranium, the tumour begins to displace tissue at first locally and then at a distance from the tumour resulting in a number of false localizing signs.

- Coma
- Unilateral, bilateral sixth nerve palsy
- Pupillary changes
- Ipsilateral or bilateral corticospinal tract signs.

4. Discuss brain edema.

Ans. i. *Vasogenic edema*: It is a type seen in the vicinity of tumour growth and other localized processes as well as more diffuse injury to the blood vessels.

   Heightened permeability in vasogenic edema is due partly to a defect in tight endothelial junctions but mainly to active vesicular transport across endothelial cells.

   The particular vulnerability of white matter to vasogenic edema may be due to less resistance to fluid under pressure than gray matter.

   ii. *Cytotoxic or cellular edema*: It occurs typically in hypoxic-ischaemic injury. It is due to failure of sodium depended ATP within cells which causes sodium accumulation followed by water and results in swelling of endothelial, glial and neuronal cells at the expense of the extracellular space of the brain.

   iii. *Interstitial edema*: It is the edema that occurs with obstructive hydrocephalus especially when the ependymal lining is lost and CSF sweeps into the periventricular tissue in the space between cells and myelin.

   Treatment of brain edema:

   - Glucocorticoids: Injection dexamathasone 4 mg sixth hourly. Useful in
     - Brain tumour
     - Brain abscess
     - Head injury

- Mannitol: 25% in a dose of 0.5 to 1 gm/kg/day in 2–10 minutes
- Controlled hyperventilation
- Dextrose solution should be avoided because of the hypo-osmolar nature.

5. What is oncogene?

Ans. The virus acts to force the cell from its normal reproductive cycle into an unrestrained replicative cycle. Because of the capacity to transform the cellular genome, the virus product is called oncogene.

6. What is hamartoma?

Ans. It is a tumour like formation that has its basis in mal-development and undergoes little change during the life of the host.

7. Discuss neuroimaging of brain tumours.

Ans. i. Brain tumours typically produce a vasogenic pattern of edema with accumulation of excess water in white matter.

ii. Contrast enhancement reflects a breakdown of the BBB (blood–brain barrier) within the tumour permitting leakage of contrast agent.

iii. Low grade gliomas typically do not exhibit contrast enhancement.

iv. Calcium is seen in CT scan in more than half of the cases of oligodendroglioma.

8. Discuss meningioma.

Ans. i. They elaborate vascular endothelial growth factor which are angiogenic and relate to both the highly vascularized nature of the tumour and their prominent surrounding edema.

ii. Some meningiomas contain estrogen and progesterone receptors and enlarge during pregnancy and are associated with breast cancer.

iii. They are extra-axial.

iv. Meningioma has a characteristic tendency to encircle one another forming whorls and psammoma bodies.

v. Usual site of meningiomas are:
- Sylvian region
- Superior parasagittal surfaces of the frontal and parietal lobes
- Olfactory groove
- Lesser wing of sphenoid bone
- Tuberculum sellar
- Superior surface of the cerebellum
- Cerebellopontine angle
- Spinal cord

vi. They have a tendency to calcify and prominent vascularity which are reflected by homogenous contrast enhancement on CT or MRI.

CT head: Dural tail: A stretch of dural enhancement flanking the main tumour mass.

9. Discuss brain metastasis?

Ans. i. 80% of the metastasis are in the cerebral hemispheres and 20% in the posterior fossa structures.

ii. Intracranial metastasis assume three main patterns
- Skull and dura
- Brain itself
- Craniospinal meninges (meningeal carcinomatosis)

iii. Predilection for the gray matter and white matter junction and for the border zone between MCA and PCA

iv. Lung is the most common site of brain metastasis

v. Stroke like episodes rather than insidious onset:
- Bleeding into the tumour
- Tumour embolism.

10. Discuss meningeal carcinomatosis.

Ans. a. Common primary sites:
- Adenocarcinoma of the breast
- Lungs

- GI tract
- Melanoma
- Childhood leukemia
- Systemic lymphoma

b. The diagnosis can be established by identifying tumour cells in CSF.

c. Polyradiculopathies, multiple cranial nerve palsies and a confusional state have been the principal manifestations.

11. What is chloroma?

Ans. In leukemia, a solid green coloured mass of mylogenous leukemic cells affecting dura and brain is called chloroma.

12. What is necrotizing leukoencephalopathy?

Ans.   i. Radiation induced white matter necrosis

ii. Radiation breaks down the BBB, allowing methotrexate to injure the myelin.

13. What are the manifestations of colloid cyst? What causes "Bobble-headed doll syndrome"?

Ans.   i. It causes an intermittent obstructive syndrome.

ii. Ball valve obstruction of the 3rd ventricle causes drop attacks.

iii. Suprasellar arachnoid cyst causes "Bobble-headed doll syndrome".

14. What are drop metastasis?

Ans. Ependymoma may metastasize via CSF pathways. Brain tumour metastasis that spread to the spinal cord by this means are termed as drop metastasis.

15. Discuss pituitary adenomas.

Ans.   i. *Microadenoma*: Tumours less than 1 cm in diameter

ii. Pituitary adenomas present with

- Endocrine abnormalities:
  - *Prolactinoma*: Treatment is bromocriptine 2.5 mgs
  - Acromegaly
  - Cushing's disease

- Visual abnormalities:
  - *Junctional scotoma*: In one eye, there is central scotoma and in the other eye, there is temporal hemianopia.
  - Bitemporal hemianopia.
iii. *Empty sella syndrome*: Non-tumorous enlargement of the sella
iv. *Pituitary apoplexy*: Result of an infarction of an adenoma that has outgrown its blood supply.

16. Discuss radiation therapy.

Ans. i. *Radiation*: Rippling (myokemia) and glucose metabolism is decreased on PET/SPECT.

Malignancy: Pain and glucose metabolism is increased on PET/SPECT.

ii. Growth hormone is the most sensitive to radiotherapy. TSH is the least sensitive.

iii. *Stereotaxis radiosurgery*: It is the administration of a focused high radiation to a precisely defined volume of tissue in a single treatment.

iv. *Interstitial brachy therapy*: It is the implantation of radioactive material into the tumour mass. It is generally reserved for tumour recurrence because of its associated toxicity.

17. Discuss acoustic neuroma (vestibular schwannoma).

Ans. i. *Types*:
  - Type I: Peripheral
  - Type II: Central: Bilateral acoustic neuromas are the hallmark
ii. Most common site 8th and 5th cranial nerves
iii. They may arise from any cranial or spinal root except the optic and olfactory nerves which are myelinated by oligodendrocytes rather than Schwann cells.
iv. Vestibular schwannomas enlarge the internal auditory canal, an imaging finding that help distinguish them from other CP angle masses.

18. Discuss neurocutaneous syndromes.

Ans. I. *Neurofibroma I*:
- Café au lait spots
- Lisch nodules (hamartoma of the iris)

II. *Tuberous sclerosis*:
- It is characterized by seizures, mental retardation, cutaneous lesions.
- *Cutaneous lesions*:
  - Adenoma sebaceum (facial angiofibromatosis)
  - Ash-leaf macules (hypopigmented)
  - Shagreen patch (yellowish thickening of the skin over the lumbosacral region).
  - Depigmented nevus

III. *Von Hippel-Lindau syndrome*:
- The syndrome consists of retinal, cerebellar and spinal hemangioblastoma which are slowly growing cystic tumours.

19. Discuss paraneoplastic disorders.

Ans. Paraneoplastic disorders are a group of neurologic disorders that occur in patients with carcinoma or some other types of neoplasam even though the nervous system is not the site of metastasis or direct invasion or direct compression of the tumour.

   i. Paraneoplastic cerebellar degeneration
   ii. Opsoclonus—myoclonus ataxic syndrome
   iii. Limb encephalitis
   iv. Paraneoplastic sensory neuronopathy
   v. Necrotizing myelopathy and subacute motor neuronopathy
   vi. Optic neuropathy
   vii. Stiff-Man syndrome
   viii. Retinopathy
   ix. Lambert-Eaten syndrome.

21 Degenerative Diseases of the Nervous System

1. What is degeneration?

Ans. It refers to a more rapid process of neuronal, myelin or tissue breakdown, the degenerative products of which evoke a more vigorous reaction of phagocytosis and cellular astrogliosis.

2. What is atrophy?

Ans. It refers to a gradual wasting and a loss of a system of neurons, leaving in their wake no degenerative products and only a sparsely cellular fibrous gliosis.

3. What are the general clinical characteristic features of degenerative diseases?

Ans. i. They tend to affect specific parts or functional systems of the nervous system

ii. Insidious onset and a slowly progressive course

iii. Irreversibility.

4. What is Capgras syndrome?

Ans. It is a delusion that a familiar person has been replaced by an impostor. Approximately 10% of Alzheimer disease patients develop Capgras syndrome.

5. What are the diagnostic criteria of Alzheimer's disease?

Ans. i. Dementia

ii. Age of patient more than 40 years

iii. Deficits in two or more areas of cognitive and progressive worsening of memory and other cognitive functions such as language, perception and motor skills (praxis)

iv. Absence of disturbed consciousness

v. Exclusion of other brain diseases.

6. What is the pathology of Alzheimer's disease?

Ans. i. The most important microscopic findings are neuritic senile plaques, neurofibrillary tangles.

ii. The accumulation of Aβ amyloid in cerebral arterioles termed as amyloid angiopathy may lead to cerebral lobe haemorrhages.

iii. Excess production of $A\beta_{42}$ is a key initiator of cellular damage in Alzheimer's disease.

iv. Adults with trisomy 21 (Down syndrome) who survive beyond age 40 constantly develop neuropathologic changes of AD.

7. What is the treatment of AD?

Ans. i. Acetylcholinesterase inhibitor, e.g. tacrine, donepezil.

ii. NMDA glutamenergic antagonist, e.g. mematine 200 mg daily.

8. Discuss Huntington's chorea.

Ans. It is a disease in which dementia is a prominent feature with other neurologic abnormalities.

• Triad of:
  – Dominant inheritance
  – Choreo—Athetosis
  – Dementia
• Usually seen in 4th and 5th decades
• Chromosome 4 and long repeat of trinucleotide (CAG)
• Frequency of blinking is increased (opposite of Parkinson's)
• Rigidity may be present (westphal)
• Characteristics are impaired initiation and slowness of the persuit and volitional saccadic movements.
• Compelled to glance at everything

- *Anticipation*: Earlier onset in successive generations
- *Pathology*: Atrophy of the head of the caudate nucleus
- Sensitive to dopamine
- *Treatment*: Dopamine antagonist—Haloperidol 10 to 20 mg.

9. Discuss dementia with lewy bodies.

Ans.
i. DLB may present in a patient with longstanding Parkinson's disease without cognitive impairment who slowly develops dementia associated with visual hallucinations, parkinsonism and fluctuating alertness.

ii. Patients with DLB are extremely sensitive to dopaminergic medications. A delirium induced by L-dopa, prescribed for parkinsonian symptoms, attributed to Parkinson's disease may be the initial clue that the correct diagnosis is DLB.

iii. α-synuclein is the main component of lewy body.

iv. *Treatment*: Anti-cholinesterase.

10. Discuss Parkinson's disease.

Ans. It is the disorder characterized by abnormal posture and movement.

i. Usual blink rate is 12 to 20 per minute but in Parkinson's disease, the blink rate is reduced to 5 to 10 per minute.

ii. Pill rolling tremor

iii. *Negroe's sign*: Cogwheel rigidity

iv. *Meyerson's sign*: Inability to inhibit blinking

v. Lewy bodies are seen in idiopathic Parkinson's disease.

vi. *Prognosis*: 7.5 to 10 years

vii. *Datatop study*: Selegiline monotherapy delays the need for levodopa therapy by 9 to 12 months

viii. *Deep brain stimulation*: Stimulation causes a functional blockade. Following DBS remaining motor system are able to compensate more effectively.

11. What are Parkinson's plus syndromes?

Ans.
i. *Progressive supranuclear palsy (Steel, Richardson Olenzewki)*: Parkinson's plus vertical gaze impairment

ii. *Shy drager syndrome*: Parkinson's plus dysautonomia (orthostatic hypotension)

iii. *Lewy body disease*: Parkinson's plus dementia

iv. *Cortico basal ganglionic degeneration*: Parkinson's plus apraxia, alien hand phenomenon is observed.

12. Discuss progressive supranuclear palsy.

Ans. i. Recurrent falls

ii. *Supranuclear ophthalmoplegia*: Difficulty in voluntary vertical movements of the eyes often downwards but sometimes upward.

iii. Pseudobulbar palsy

iv. Axial dystonia.

13. Discuss multi-system atrophy (MSA).

Ans. *Types*:

- Striatonigral degeneration
- Olivopontocerebellar degeneration
- Shy-Drager syndrome

Features:

- Lack of response to L-dopa
- Absence of tremor
- Symmetry of signs
- Presence of autonomic disorder, cerebellar and Parkinson's features.

14. Discuss L-dopa.

Ans. Side-effects:

- On-off phenomenon
- Dyskinetic movements

  Mechanism: Denervation supersensitivity

Treatment of L-dopa induced side-effects:

- Use of lower dose of long acting preparation
- Amantidine
- Clozapine
- Low protein diet (based on the notion that alimentary derived amino acids antagonize the clinical effects of L-dopa).

15. What is bradyphrenia?

Ans. It is the cognitive equivalent of bradykinesia.

16. What is Segawa syndrome (juvenile-dystonia-parkinsonian syndrome)?

Ans. i. Disappears during sleep, diurinal variation
ii. Response to L-dopa 10 mg/kg/day.

17. What is the syndrome of progressive blindness?

Ans. i. Hereditary optic atrophy of leber
ii. Retinitis pigmentosa.

18. What is Meig's syndrome?

Ans. It is the combination of lower facial and jaw dystonia.

19. How does botulinum toxin act?

Ans. Botulinum toxin acts by blocking the release of acetylcholine at the neuromuscular junction resulting in dose dependent weakness.

20. What is normal pressure hydrocephalus (NPH)?

Ans. It is a triad of:
- Abnormal gait
- Dementia
- Urinary incontinence

Investigation: Radionuclide cisternography shows the delay in CSF absorption over the convexity.

21. What is Marchiafava-Bignami disease?

Ans. A rare syndrome of dementia along with seizures with degeneration of the corpus callosum has been reported primarily in male Italian drinkers of red wine.

22. What is Wernicke's encephalopathy?

Ans. Thiamine (vitamin B_1) deficiency in a malnourished individual (frequently but not necessarily alcoholic) with confusion, ataxia and diplopia from ophthalmoplegia.

23. What is motor neuron disease?

Ans. i. Degenerative disease affecting only motor pathways

ii. *Mill's variant*: Only hemiplegia is seen

iii. *Treatment*:

Riluzole: It may reduce excitotoxicity by diminishing glutamate release.

iv. May need ventilator support if there is respiratory insufficiency.

Vital capacity: Deep breath count multiplied by 100 is the vital capacity.

e.g. 25 × 100 = 2.5 litres is the vital capacity.

24. What are the heredofamilial forms of progressive muscular atrophy?

Ans. i. *Werdnig-Hoffmann type*: After cystic fibrosis, this is the most frequent cause of death of a recessively inherited disease (preterm to six months).

ii. *Kugelberg-Welander type*: (One year to adolescence).

iii. *Kennedy syndrome (bulbospinal atrophy)*: Early adulthood, an unusual pattern of distal muscular atrophy with prominent bulbar signs with gynecomastia.

iv. *Fazio-Londe disease*: Progressive bulbar palsy of childhood.

25. Discuss syndrome of progressive ataxia.

Ans. 1. *Fredrich's ataxia*:
- Accounts for about half of all cases of hereditary ataxias
- Chromosome 9 (frataxin protein)
- Hammer toes, cardiomyopathy and diabetes mellitus
- *Static ataxia*: Ataxia on standing
- Posterior column: Romberg's sign is present.
- *Treatment*: Oral 5 hyroxytryptophan

2. *Olivopontocerebellar atrophy (OPCA)*: Cerebellar atrophy with brain stem signs

3. *Cerebellar atrophy with predominantly basal ganglionic features*:
- Machado-Joseph disease.
- DRPLA (dentatorubropallidolysian atrophy): Chorea is associated.

4. Paroxysmal ataxias.

22

Spinal Cord Disorders

1. What are the types of spinal injuries?

Ans. i. Fracture dislocation

ii. Pure fracture

iii. Pure dislocation

iv. Ratio of 3:1:1.

2. What are the clinical effects of spinal cord injury?

Ans. i. All voluntary movements below the lesion are lost.

ii. Sensations are abolished.

iii. Spinal shock (1–6 weeks): Tendon and autonomic reflexes are lost.

Bullbocavernous reflex is the first to return.

3. What is the mechanism of spinal shock?

Ans. It is due to sudden interruption of suprasegmental descending fibre system (facilitatory tracts–reticulospinal and vestibulospinal tracts) that normally keeps the spinal motor neurons in a continuous state of sublimal depolarization (ready to respond).

4. What are the stages of heightened reflex activity?

Ans. i. Usually after a few weeks, the reflex response to stimulation which are initially minimal and unsustained, becomes stronger and more easily elicitable and as time passes comes to include additional and more proximal muscles.

ii. *Mass reflex*:

- This can be evoked by stimulation of the skin of the legs or by some interoceptive stimulus such as full bladder.
- *Occurs after several months*: The withdrawal reflex becomes greatly exaggerated to the point of flexor spasms and may be accompanied by profuse sweating, piloerection, automatic emptying of the bladder (occasionally of the rectum).

iii. *Autonomic dysreflexia*: Below the level absence of sweating, above the level exaggerated sweating.

iv. *Paraplegia in flexion*: Seen in complete lesions.

Paraplegia in extension: Seen in partial lesions (extra pyramidal tracts which maintain extension posture are spared). Has better prognosis.

v. *Cruciate paralysis*:

- Weakness is practically limited to the arms.
- Attributable to the segregation of the corticospinal fibers to the arm (rostral) and to the legs (caudal) within the pyramidal decussation.
- Seen in patients who survive injuries of the very rostral cervical cord.

5. What is the relationship of the spinal roots to the vertebral bodies?

Ans. i. C_1–C_7 (cervical roots) exit through foramina above their respective vertebral bodies, e.g. C_7 root above C_7 body.

ii. C_8 exits above T_1, e.g. C_8 root above T_1 body.

iii. Other roots (T_1 and below) exit and issue below other bodies, e.g. T_1 below T_1 vertebral body.

6. Where does spinal cord infarction occur?

Ans. With systemic hypotension cord, infarction occurs at the level of greatest ischaemic risks often T_3–T_4 and also at the boundary zones between the anterior and posterior spinal artery territories.

7. What is Beevor's sign?

Ans. Lesions at T_9–T_{10} paralyze the lower but not the upper abdominal muscles, resulting in upward movement of the umbilicus when the abdominal wall contracts.

8. What is the treatment of spinal cord injury?

Ans.   i. Immobilisation of cervical spine

    ii. Methylpredisolone below 30 mg/kg followed by 5.4 mg/kg/hour.

  iii. The prognosis for recovery is more favorable if any movement or sensation is elicitable during the first 48 to 72 hours.

9. What is the treatment of bladder disorders?

Ans.   i. *Treatment of detrusor spasticity*: Anticholinergic drug: Imipramine 25 to 200 mg/day.

    ii. *Treatment for sphincter to relax during bladder emptying*: Terazosine (α-adrenergic blocking agent) 1 to 2 gm tid.

10. What is the treatment of spasticity?

Ans. *Baclofen (15 to 240 mg)*: It acts by facilitating GABA mediated inhibition of motor reflex arc.

11. Discuss myelitis.

Ans. *Acute*: Days to 2 weeks

Subacute: 2 weeks to 6 weeks

Chronic: More than 6 weeks

Myelitis due to multiple sclerosis and post-infectious process will be found to be the most common cause in practice.

12. When does cervical spondylotic changes manifest?

Ans.   i. Normal canal diameter is 17 to 18 mm.

    ii. Cervical spondylotic occurs when it is 7 to 12 mm.

13. Discuss craniovertebral anomalies.

Ans.   i. Fusion of the atlas and foramen magnum is the most common.

   ii. Atlantoaxial dislocation (atlas displaced anteriorly in relation to axis)
  iii. Absence of odontoid
  iv. *Klippel-Feil syndrome*: Fusion of the upper cervical vertebra or atlas to the occiput
   v. *Platybasia*: Flattening of the base of the skull (the angle formed by intersection of the plane of the clivus and the plane of anterior fossae is greater than 135 degrees
  vi. *Basilar impression or invagination*: Upward bulging of the occipital condyles above the plane of the foramen magnum.

14. What is the MRI appearance of spinal arachnoiditis?

Ans. *MRI*: Candle-guttering appearance.

15. What is the characteristic feature of intraspinal tumours?

Ans. In distinction to brain tumours, the majority of intraspinal tumours are benign and produce the effects mainly by compression of the spinal cord rather than by ischaemia.

16. What are the various spinal tumours?

Ans. Most common primary extramedullary tumours are Neurofibroma and meningioma. Together they form 55% of tumours. Intramedullary are ependymoma (60%) and astrocytoma (25%).

17. Differentiate between intramedullary and extramedullary syndromes.

Ans. *Intramedullary syndrome*:
   • The pathology is within the substance of the cord.
   • Intramedullary lesions tend to produce poorly localized burning pain rather than radicular pain and spare sensation in the perianal and sacral areas (sacral sparing) reflecting the laminated configuration of the spinothalamic tract with sacral fibres outermost, corticospinal tract signs appear later.
   Extramedullary syndrome:
   • The pathology is outside the substance of the cord, compresses the spinal cord or its vascular supply.

- The radicular pain is often prominent and there is early sacral sensory loss (lateral spinothalamic tract) and spastic weakness in the legs (corticospinal tract) due to superficial location of leg fibres in the corticospinal tract. Further distinction is made between extradural and intradural masses, as the former are generally malignant and the later benign. A long duration of symptoms favors an intradural origin.

18. What is dissociated sensory loss?

Ans. i. Dissociated sensory loss is recognizable by loss of pain and temperature sensation with sparing of touch and vibration. It is because only the crossing spinothalamic tracts fibers get affected with sparing of posterior column tract.

ii. Characteristically seen in syringomyelia.

19. What is Barnette's classification of syringomyelia?

Ans. *Type I*: Syringomyelia with obstruction of the foramen magnum. Type I chiari malformation may be associated
Type II: Syringomyelia without obstruction of the foramen magnum
Type III: Syringomyelia with other diseases of the spinal cord
Type IV: Pure hydromyelia.

20. What does Babinski sign indicate?

Ans. Babinski sign indicates that the spinal cord is involved above the fifth lumbar segment.

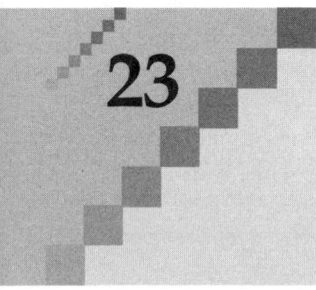

23 Peripheral Nerve Disorders

1. What are segmental demyelination, wallerian degeneration and axonal degeneration?

Ans. *Segmental demyelination*: Focal degeneration of myelin sheath and sparing of the axon
Wallerian degeneration: Dying forward
Axonal degeneration: Dying backward (distal most site to proximal site).

2. Discuss small fibre neuropathy (painful neuropathies and dissociated sensory loss).

Ans. i. Diminished pinprick and temperature sensations often with painful and burning dysesthesias
  ii. Autonomic dysfunction
  iii. Relative sparing of motor power, balance and tendon jerks
  iv. Tendon reflexes may sometimes be retained because afferent arc of the tendon reflexes utilizes the large heavily myelinated fibres.
  Examples: Lepromatous leprosy, diabetes.

3. Discuss large fibre neuropathy (ataxic neuropathies).

Ans. i. Motor dysfunction, sensory ataxia, areflexia
  ii. Minor cutaneous sensory deficits
  iii. Loss of sensory functions that are dependent on large fibres in the presence of preserved reflexes implicate the central projection of sensory ganglion cells, i.e. a lesion in the posterior column of the spinal cord.
  Example: Vitamin B_{12} neuropathy.

4. What are the signs of autonomic neuropathy?

Ans. 1. *Mainly negative*: (Loss of function)
- Postural hypotension
- Anhidrosis
- Hypothermia
- Bladder atony
- Obstipation
- Dry mouth
- Blurring of vision from lack of pupillary responses
- Sexual impotence

2. *Positive phenomenon (hyperfunction)*:
- Episodic hypertension
- Diarrhea
- Hyperhidrosis
- Tachycardia or bradycardia

3. *Types*:
- Acute: GBS
- Chronic: Diabetes.

5. Discuss thickening of nerves in relation to disease patterns.

Ans. i. *Leprous neuritis*: Fusiform thickening of nerve trunks
ii. *Amyloid polyneuropathy*: Beading of nerve trunks
iii. *Genetically determined hypertrophic neuropathies*: Uniform thickening of all nerve trunks.

6. What is mononeuropathy multiplex (multifocal neuropathy)?

Ans. i. Mononeuropathy multiplex refers to simultaneous or sequential involvement of individual noncontiguous nerve trunks.
ii. One-third is due to demyelination.
iii. Two-thirds are due to axonal which is due to predominantly ischaemic (vasculitis: PAN [renal and bowel involvement takes place, P-ANCA is positive], Churg-Strauss disease [Lung and skin involvement takes place, C-ANCA is present in Wegner's granulomatosis and Churg-Strauss diseases]).

7. What are the important features of radiculopathy?

Ans. i. Regional loss of a reflex is a sign of radiculopathy.

ii. Preservation of sensory potentials in nerves that innervate regions of sensory loss and supply weak and denervated muscles.

iii. Loss of F and H late responses

iv. Weakness and denervation in the
   a. Paraspinal
   b. Gluteal
   c. Rhomboid muscles
   which are supplied by nerves that arise very proximally from the roots.

8. What are the features of claw foot?

Ans. a. Dorsiflexion of proximal phalanges

b. Plantar flexion of distal phalanges

c. Shortening of the foot

d. Heightening of the arch.

9. What causes kyphoscoliosis?

Ans. Unequal weakening of paravertebral muscles on the two sides of the spine.

10. What is Tinel's phenomenon?

Ans. Generation of a tingling sensation in the sensory territory of the nerve by tapping along the course of the nerve trunk.

11. What is hyperpathia?

Ans. Light stimuli to hypesthetic areas, once perceived may be experienced as extremely uncomfortable.

12. Discuss nerve conduction studies.

Ans. 1. *Demyelination*:
   - Slowing of nerve conduction velocity
   - Dispersion of evoked compound action potentials

- Conduction block (major decrease in amplitude of muscle compound action potentials on proximal stimulation of the nerve as compared to distal stimulation)
  - Marked prolongation of distal latencies
2. *Axonal*: A reduction in amplitude of evoked compound action potentials with relative preservation of nerve conduction velocity.

13. Discuss EMG findings of myopathic disorders and neuropathic disorders.

Ans. Normal muscle potentials appear as waveforms with a duration of 5–15 ms, 2–4 phases and amplitudes of 0.5–3 mV.

1. *Myopathic disorders*: Small, short duration polyphasic muscle action potentials recruited in excessive numbers for a given degree of voluntary muscle contraction.
2. *Neuropathic disorders*:
   a. *Reinnervation*: Large and polyphasic motor unit potentials
   b. *Deinnervation*: Features a decrease in the number of motor units activated by maximal effort to contract muscle but an increase in the rate of firing of the remaining motor units
      - *Fibrillation*: Random, unregulated firing of individual denervated muscle fibres
      - *Fasciculation*: Random, spontaneous firing of motor units which in chronic state can be markedly enlarged and polyphasic
      - Positive sharp waves
      - Complex repetitive discharges.

14. Discuss Guillain-Barré syndrome.

Ans. i. Guillain-Barré Syndrome (GBS) is an acute, frequently severe, and fulminant polyradiculoneuropathy that is autoimmune in nature.

 ii. Facial diparesis is present in 50% of affected individuals.

 iii. *Miller Fisher syndrome*:
   - It is seen in 5% of all GBS patients.

- Triad of
  - Ophthalmoplegia
  - Ataxia
  - Areflexia
- *Anti-GQ1b antibodies (90%)*: They are not found in other forms of GBS unless there is extraocular motor nerve involvement.
iv. Anti-ganglioside antibodies most frequently to GM1 are common in GBS (20 to 50%) particularly in those preceded by C. Jejuni infection.
v. *Immunotherapy*:
  - 2 weeks after the first motor symptoms, immunotherapy is no longer effective.
  - IVIg is administered as five daily infusions for a total of 2 gm per kg (0.4 gm/kg/daily for five days).
  - There is some evidence that GBS auto-antibodies are neutralized by anti-idiotypic antibodies present in IVIg preparations perhaps accounting for the therapeutic effect.
  - 30% of the GBS patients require ventilatory support.
  - CIDP is differentiated from GBS by:
    - Prolonged and relapsing course (8 or 12 weeks)
    - Enlargement of nerves
    - Responsiveness to corticosteroids.

15. Discuss diabetic neuropathy.

Ans. i. 15% have symptoms and 50% have evidence of diabetic neuropathy by nerve conduction studies.
ii. *Diabetic mononeuropathy*:
  - Painful 3rd nerve palsy with sparing of pupillary functions (because parasympathetic fibres run superficially on the 3rd nerve. Hence, in diabetic neuropathy which affects the centre of the nerve, parasympathetic fibers are not affected, whereas in compressive 3rd nerve lesions like posterior communicating artery aneurysms and subdural haematomas, the superficially placed parasympathetic fibres get affected resulting in pupillary dilatation).
  - Femoral, sciatic and peroneal nerve may get affected.

iii. *Diabetic autonomic neuropathy*: Severe abdominal and limb pain.
iv. *Diabetic amyotrophy (asymmetric proximal motor neuropathy)*: The most evident features are weakened muscles innervated by the femoral and obturator nerves (quadriceps, iliopsoas, adductor magnus) and ipsilateral loss of knee jerk reflex.
v. *Aldose reductase inhibitors*: The role of aldose reductase inhibitors in preventing or reversing diabetic complications including neuropathy remains unclear.

16. Discuss hereditary neuropathies.

Ans. i. The characteristic feature of hereditary neuropathies are uniformity of electrophysiologic changes.
ii. *Classification*:
- HMSN-I/CMT-I: Demyelination, enlarged nerves (greater auricular nerve), nerve conduction velocity is decreased, onion bulb appearance, PMP_{22}.
- HMSN-II/CMT-II: Axonal (P_0)
- HMSN-III: Dejerine-Sottas disease
- HMSN-IV: Refsum disease
  - Retinitis pigmentosa (night blindness)
  - Cerebellar ataxia
  - Neuropathy: Phytanic acid levels are increased.

17. What are the inherited polyneuropathies with a recognized metabolic disorder?

Ans. 1. *Refsum's disease*:
2. *Abetalipoprotinemia (Bassen-Kornzweig syndrome)*:
- Acanthocytosis
- Cerebellar features, neuropathy
- Low serum cholesterol
3. *Tangier's disease*:
- Atherosclerosis
- Yellow-orange tonsils
- Neuropathy (pain and temperature are decreased)
4. *Fabry's disease*: Angiokeratoma corporis diffusm.

18. What is hereditary neuropathy with liability to pressure palsies?

Ans. HNPP (also called tomaccous neuropathy) is an autosommal dominant disorder that produces an episodic demyelinating neuropathy.

19. What is POEMS syndrome?

Ans. Polyneuropathy
Organomegaly
Endocrinopathy
Mprotein and
Skin changes are seen in multiple myeloma.

20. What is Bing-Neel syndrome?

Ans. A significant proportion of patients with waldenstorn macroglobulinemia have a hyperviscosity state manifested by diffuse slowing of retinal and cerebral circulation giving rise to episodic confusion, coma, impairment of vision and sometimes stroke.

21. What is MGUS (monoclonal gammopathy of undetermined significance)?

Ans. Monoclonal proteins underlie the largest group of otherwise unexplained neuropathies in adults.

22. What is the treatment of porphyric polyneuropathy?

Ans. *Treatment*: Intravenous glucose (4 mg/kg for 3 to 14 days) to suppress the heme biosynthetic pathway.

23. What is the effect of thallium?

Ans. It causes rapid hair loss.

24. What causes sensory neuronopathy?

Ans. Small cell cancer of the lung: Anti-Hu antibody.

25. What is the treatment of INH induced neuropathy?

Ans. 150 to 450 mg of pyridoxine daily.

26. What is the clinical presentation of herpes zoster?

Ans.　i. Ophthalmoplegic zoster

　　　ii. Ramsay Hunt syndrome.

27. What are the sites and clinical features of leprous neuritis?

Ans.　i. It usually affects cool parts.

　　　ii. Tendon reflexes are usually preserved because of the sparing of most of the muscular and larger sensory nerves.

　　　iii. It is one exception to the rule that all chronic neuropathies are more or less symmetrical in pattern.

28. What is the triad of Lyme disease?

Ans.　i. Cranial nerve palsies

　　　ii. Radiculitis

　　　iii. Aseptic meningitis.

29. What are the differentiating points between radiation plexopathy and tumour plexopathy?

Ans.　i. *Radiation plexopathy*: Upper plexus are involved, myokymea and fasciculation.

　　　ii. *Tumour plexopathy*: Lower plexus are involved.

30. Differentiate between abduction weakness of median nerve and radial nerve.

Ans.　*Median nerve*: Abduction of the thumb in the plane at a right angle to the palm is affected (abductor and flexor policies brevis). *Radial nerve*: Abduction of the thumb in the plane of the palm is affected.

31. Discuss carpal tunnel syndrome.

Ans.　i. It is an entrapment neuropathy of median nerve.

　　　ii. Dysesthesias may be prominent at night but absent during the day.

　　　iii. Provocative tests:

　　　　　a. *Phalen maneuver*: Consists of hyperflexion of the wrist for 30 to 60 seconds usually performed by opposing the outer surface of the hands and wrists flexed.

b. *Tinel sign*: It is elicited by lightly tapping the volar aspect of the wrist at the transverse carpal ligament.

Both of these tests are meant to elicit pain or paraesthesias over the digits innervated by the median nerve.

iv. *Treatment*: Splinting of the wrist to avoid flexion almost always relieves the discomfort but denies the patient the full use of hand for sometime.

32. Differentiate between metastasis and radiation affecting lumbosacral plexus?

Ans. Metastasis causes pain

Radiation causes weakness.

33. What are the important investigations of neuropathy?

Ans. i. Blood sugar level

ii. Serum protein electrophoresis

iii. Nerve conduction studies

iv. Nerve biopsy.

34. What are the indications of nerve biopsy?

Ans. i. Mononeuritis multiplex

ii. Genetically determined childhood disorders such as metachromatic leukodystrophy.

35. What biopsy is done in Sjögren sicca syndrome?

Ans. Lip biopsy.

24 Myasthenia Gravis, Muscle and Related Disorders

1. What is myasthenia gravis?

Ans. Myasthenia gravis (MG) is a neuromuscular disorder characterized by weakness and fatigability of skeletal muscles.

2. What are the characteristic features of myasthenia gravis?

Ans. Combined weakness of the extraocular muscles (levator and orbicularis oculi) with normal pupillary response to light and accommodation is virtually diagnostic of myasthenia.

3. What is myasthenic crisis?

Ans. i. If weakness of respiration becomes so severe as to require respiratory assistance, the patient is said to be in crisis.

ii. Intercurrent infection is the most common cause of myasthenic crisis.

4. Classify myasthenia.

Ans. i. Ocular myasthenia: 20%

ii. a. Mild generalized myasthenia: 25%

b. Moderate generalized myasthenia: 25%

iii. Acute and respiratory crisis: 20%

iv. Late severe myasthenia: 20%.

5. Describe RNS (repetitive nerve stimulation).

Ans. i. Anti-AchE medication is stopped 6 to 24 hours before testing.

ii. *Electric shocks*: 2 to 3 per second to the appropriate nerves.

13. Describe congenital neuromuscular disorders.

Ans. The characteristic feature of most of these myopathies is lack of progression or extremely slow progression. They are:
- Central core disease (every patient is a potential candidate for the development of malignant hyperthermia).
- Nemaline rod myopathy
- Myotubular myopathy
- Myofibrillar myopathy.

14. What are sodium channel disorders?

Ans. i. *Hyperkalemic periodic paralysis*: Weakness appearing after a period of rest that follows exercise is particularly characteristic.

ii. *Paragyotonia congenital*:
   a. Cold exaggerates myotonia.
   b. This is in contrast to classic myotonia which alleviates the condition.

15. What are the disorders of the calcium channel?

Ans. a. *Hypokalemic periodic paralysis*:
- It is never seen after 25 years of age except thyrotoxic periodic paralysis.
- Presumably large quantities of potassium enter the muscle fibres during an attack.
- *Prophylaxis* : Acetazolamide 250 mg three times daily may work through the production of acidosis.
- *Treatment*: Low carbohydrate, low salt, decrease in exercise
   – Potassium: 0.2 to 0.4 mm/kg every 30 minutes orally.
   – IV potassium in mannitol if necessary .

b. *Malignant hyperthermia*:
- Interference in relaxation of muscle
- IV dantrolene 1 mg/kg.

16. What are potassium channel disorders?

Ans. Anderson's syndrome (episodic weakness, dysmorphic features).

17. What are chloride channel disordes?

Ans. *Autosomal dominant*: Thomsen disease
Autosomal recessive: Myotonia worsened by cold and improved by exercise
Treatment: Phenytoin.

18. Correlate muscle weakness with clinical effects.

Ans. i. *Weakness of gluteus muscles*: Waddling gait
ii. *Weakness of ileopsoas and abdominal muscles*: Lumbar lordosis
iii. *Asymmetrical weakness of paravertebal muscles*: Kyphoscoliosis
iv. *Fibrous contracture of calf muscle*: Equinovarous deformities
v. *Weakness of trapezius/serratus muscles*: Flaring of shoulders blades.

19. What is Gower's sign?

Ans. *Gower's sign*: This term describes the maneuver of rising from a supine position in the presence of marked proximal weakness. The patient must roll to a prone position, push off the floor, lock the knees and push the upper body upward by *climbing up* the legs with the hands. Although Gower's sign is associated with myopathies, it is present in any patient with marked proximal weakness.

20. What is arthrogryposis (multiplex congenita)?

Ans. i. Fibrous contractures involving multiple muscle groups
ii. Syndrome of newborn:
   • An onset during intrauterine life
   • Attenuation of the neural or muscular apparatus that results in muscular weakness
iii. Contracture and fixity of the limbs in arthrogryposis are the results of immobility of developing joints consequent upon muscle weakness during fetal development.

21. What is myotonia?

Ans. A condition of prolonged muscle contraction followed by slow muscle relaxation.

Examples:
- Myotonia congenita, paramyotonia congenita
- In myotonic dystrophy, there are facial weakness and ptosis.

22. What is the peculiarity of ocular muscles?

Ans. In ocular muscles, a motor unit contains only 6–10 muscle fibres whereas gastronemus contains 1800 fibres. Therefore, pathological disorders easily manifest in ocular muscles clinically.

23. What is second-wind phenomenon?

Ans. Exercise tolerance can be enhanced by a slow induction phase (warm-up) or brief periods of rest allowing for the start of the second-wind phenomenon (switching to utilization of fatty acids).

24. What is forearm ischaemic test?

Ans. Generally in ischaemia, the lactate rises, but in patients with McArdle and Taurus disease, the lactate fails to rise.

25. Discuss inflammatory myopathies.

Ans. i. Inflammation is the histologic hallmark of the disease.

ii. *Types*:
- *Polymyositis*: Connective tissue disorder and auto-immune disorders are frequent.
- *Dermatomyositis*:
  - Malignancy
  - Rash
- *Heliotrope*: Eye
- *Gottrom*: Knuckles
- *Inclusion body myositis*:
  - Seen in more than 50 years of age
  - Weakness and atrophy of distant muscles
  - IBM has the least favourable prognosis of the inflammatory myopathies.

iii. *Treatment*: Steroids, immunosuppressive drugs.

26. What are hereditary myopathies?

Ans. It refers to a group of hereditary progressive disease each with unique phenotype and genetic pattern.
- *Duchene*: Unable to walk after age 12.
- *Becker*: Able to walk after age 15.
- *Outliers*: Intermediate between Duchene and Becker.

27. What are mitochondrial myopathies?

Ans. Mitochondrial genes are derived almost exclusively from the mother accounting for the maternal inheritance of mitochondrial disorders
  a. Chronic progressive external ophthalmoplegia
  b. MERRF, melas
  c. Pure myopathy syndrome.

28. What are the features of hypothyroidism?

Ans. i. *Hoffmann syndrome*: Prominent muscle enlargement, weakness and muscle stiffness
  ii. Muscle stretch reflexes prolonged in 25% of cases.

29. What is glucocorticoid related myopathy?

Ans. i. Chronic use of prednisolone at a daily dose of more than 30 mg per day is often associated with toxicity.
  ii. Muscle biopsy in chronic cases show preferential type 2 muscle fibre atrophy.

25 Molecular Biology, Clinical Study and Investigations

1. What are gated ion channels?

Ans. Most ion channels are gated, meaning that they can transit between confirmations that are open or closed to ion conductance.

2. What are ionotropic and metabotropic receptors?

Ans. *Ionotropic receptors*: They are direct ion channels that open after engagement by the neurotransmitter.
Metabotropic receptors: They interact with G proteins, stimulating production of second messengers and activating protein kinase which modulate a variety of cellular events.

3. What is the mechanism of addictive drugs?

Ans. Addictive drugs share the property of increasing dopamine release in the nucleus accumbens.

4. What is the correlation between cell death and NMDA receptors?

Ans. The distribution of cells sensitive to ischaemia corresponds closely with that of NMDA receptors (except for cerebellar Purkinje cells which are vulnerable to hypoxia-ischaemia but lack NMDA receptors).

5. What is apoptosis (programmed cell death)?

Ans. i. Apoptosis is favoured under conditions in which ATP levels are present.
ii. The best characterized genetic neurologic disorder related to apoptosis is infantile spinal muscular atrophy (Werdnig-Hoffmann disease).

6. What is the relevance of permeability transition pore?

Ans. Blocking the mitochondrial pore reduces both hypoglycemic and ischaemic cell death.

7. What is neurodegeneration?

Ans.　i. Protein aggregation is a major histopathologic hallmark of neurodegenerative disease.

　　ii. An inability to degrade protein aggregates could lead to cellular dysfunction, impaired axonal transport and cell death by apoptic mechanism.

8. What is blood–brain barrier (BBB)?

Ans. Astrocytic foot process that encircles the subendothelial basal surface of small blood vessels in the brain contribute to development and maintenance of BBB.

9. What is blood nerve barrier?

Ans.　i. In contrast to BBB in the PNS, the blood nerve barrier is incomplete.

　　ii. Endothelial tight junctions are lacking and the capacity of charged molecules including antibiotics to cross the barrier appears to be greatest in two regions of the PNS.

　　　• Proximally in the spinal roots, e.g. GBS

　　　• Distally at the neuromuscular junction, e.g. myasthenia gravis.

10. What are the major antigen presenting cells?

Ans.　i. Microglial cells

　　ii. Macrophages.

11. What are the manifestations of primary neuronal (gray matter) disorders?

Ans.　i. Cognitive disturbances

　　ii. Movement disorders

　　iii. Seizures.

12. What are white matter disorders?

Ans. It is a disorder of long tracts:
   i. Motor
   ii. Sensory
   iii. Visual
   iv. Cerebellar pathways.

13. What is a Lhermitte symptom?

Ans. Electric shock like sensations evoked by neck flexion is due to ectopic impulse generation in white matter pathways and occurs with demyelination in the cervical spinal cord.

14. What is the significance of temporal course of neurological illness?

Ans. i. Rapid onest of a neurological complaint:
   • Vascular
   • Seizures
   • Migraine
   ii. A gradual evolution of symptoms over hours or days:
   • Toxic
   • Metabolic
   • Infections
   • Inflammatory process
   iii. Slowly progressive:
   • Degenerative
   • Chronic infections
   • Gradual intoxications
   • Neoplasms.

15. What is the importance of family history?

Ans. i. Huntington's disease.
   ii. Charcot-Marie tooth disease.

16. What is the sign of potential weakness?

Ans. Pronator weakness especially if asymmetric is a sign of potential weakness.

17. What is pyramidal weakness?

Ans. Unilateral or bilateral weakness of the upper limb extensors and lower limb flexors (pyramidal weakness) suggests a lesion of the pyramidal tract.

18. Enumerate higher functions.

Ans.
a. Level of consciousness
b. Orientation
c. Speech and language
d. Memory
e. Fund of information
f. Unsight
g. Judgement
h. Abstract thought
i. Calculation.

19. What is Jendrassik maneuver?

Ans. Reflexes may be enhanced by asking the patient to voluntarily contract other distal muscle groups.
Examples:
• Upper limb reflexes may be reinforced by voluntary teeth clenching.
• Achilles reflex by hooking the flexed fingers of the two hands together and attempting to pull them apart.

20. What is the grading of reflexes?

Ans. 0 = Absent
1 = Present but diminished
2 = Normoactive
3 = Exaggerated
4 = Clonus.

21. What is Bayes theorem?

Ans. One is more likely to encounter rare manifestations of common diseases than the typical manifestations of rare diseases.

22. What is electroencephalography?

Ans. The electroencephalography records spontaneous electrical activity generated in the cerebral cortex.
There are four types of waves:
- *Alpha waves*: 8–12 per second 50 mv sinusoidal waves
- *Beta waves*: Faster than 12 Hz and of lower amplitude (10–20 mv)
- *Theta waves*: 4–7 Hz
- *Delta waves*: 1–3 Hz activity; is not present in the normal waking adult.

23. What are evoked potentials?

Ans. The stimulation of sense organs or peripheral nerves evokes an electrical response in the corresponding cortical receptive areas and in a number of subcortical relay stations.
The evoked potentials are useful in diagnosing disorders even before they are clinically manifested.

24. What is diffusion MR?

Ans. A sequence that detects reduction of microscopic motion of water is the most sensitive technique for detecting acute ischaemic stroke and is useful in the detection of encephalitis, abscess and prion disease.

25. What is attenuation in CT scan?

Ans. Greater X-ray attenuation, e.g. as caused by bone results in high density while soft tissue structures which have poor attenuation of X-rays are lower in density.

26. What is contrast enhancement?

Ans. i. In the normal CNS, only vessels and structures lacking a BBB, i.e.
    a. Pituitary gland
    b. Choroid plexus
    c. Dura enhance after contrast administration
  ii. Pathologically
    a. Tumour
    b. Infarcts
    c. Infections enhance.

27. What is contrast nephropathy?

Ans. i. It may result from:

a. Heamodynamic changes

b. Renal tubular obstruction

c. Cell damage

d. Immunological reactions to contrast agents

ii. Non-ionic agents and good hydration are safer.

28. What is the significance of various signal intensities (T_1, T_2 wt images)?

Ans. i. Fat and subacute haemorrhages have a high signal intensity on T_1 wt image.

ii. Structures containing more water such as CSF and edema have low signal intensity on T_1 wt image and a high signal intensity on T_2 wt image.

iii. a. T_1 wt image is more sensitive to

i. Subacute haemorrhage

ii. Fat containing structures

b. T_2 wt images are more sensitive to

i. Edema

ii. Demyelination

iii. Infarction

iv. Chronic haemorrhage

iv. Gray matter contains 10–15% more water than white matter which accounts for much of the contrast on MRI.

29. What is flair?

Ans. i. Fluid attenuated inversion recovery is a useful pulse sequence that produce T_2 wt image in which the normal high signal intensity of CSF is suppressed.

ii. Flair images are more sensitive than standard spin echo images for the detection of lesions within or adjacent to CSF.

30. What is gradient echo imaging?

Ans. It is the most sensitive to magnetic susceptibility as seen with

   i. Blood

   ii. Calcium

   iii. Air

   and is indicated in patients with traumatic brain injury.

31. What is MR contrast material (gadolinium-DTPA)?

Ans. i. Gadolinium-DTPA is a paramagnetic substance which means that it reduces the T_1 and T_2 relaxation times of water protons resulting in a high signal of T_1 wt images and a low signal on T_2 w images.

   ii. Gadolinium-DTPA does not cross the intact BBB but will enhance lesion lacking a BBB.

32. What is magnetic resonance angiography?

Ans. i. MRA has proved useful in evaluation of the extracranial carotid and vertebral circulation as well as of large calibre intracranial arteries and dural sinuses.

   ii. It has also proved useful in the non-invasive detection of intracranial aneurysms and vascular malformations.

33. What is the diffusion perfusion mismatch (echo planar MR imaging)?

Ans. *Diffusion perfusion mismatch*: The discrepancy between the region of poor perfusion and the diffusion deficit is called diffusion perfusion mismatch and is a measure of ischaemic penumbra.

Diffusion perfusion mismatch is useful in:

   a. Ischaemic penumbra

   b. Encephalitis

   c. Abscess.

34. What is functional MRI?

Ans. i. Functional MRI of the brain is an EPI technique that localizes region of activity in the brain following task activation.

    ii. The technique has proved useful to neuroscientists interested in interrogating the localization of certain brain functions.

35. What are the normal and abnormal CSF pressures?

Ans. i. *Normal*: 100 to 180 mm of water (adults)

    ii. *Children*: 30 to 60 mm of water

    iii. Increased intracranial pressure: Above 200 mm of water

    iv. Intracranial hypotension: Below 50 mm of water.

36. What is the normal cellularity of CSF?

Ans. *Normally*: No cells or at the most up to five lymphocytes.

37. Discuss proteins of CSF.

Ans. i. *Normal*: 45 mg/dl

    ii. *Viral infection*: Mainly lymphocytic reaction and a lesser elevation of protein

    iii. *Froin's syndrome*: Indicates CSF block where

        a. Protein value is more than 1000 mg

        b. CSF is deeply yellow and readily clots because of the presence of fibrinogen.

38. Discuss glucose in CSF.

Ans. i. Normal: 45 to 80 mg/dl, i.e. about two thirds of that in blood.

    ii. *Equilibration*: After the intravenous injection of glucose, 2 to 4 hrs are required to reach equilibrium with CSF.

    iii. Hypoglycorrhachia (low value of CSF glucose)

        a. Pyogenic

        b. Tuberculosis

        c. Fungal meningitis

    iv. *Viral infections*: Do not lower CSF glucose.

39. What is post-lumbar puncture headache?

Ans. i. It is seen in one-third of patients.

    ii. The pain is presumably the result of a reduction of CSF pressure and tugging on cerebral and dural vessels as the patient assumes the erect posture.

40. How does mannitol reduce edema?

Ans. i. As the osmolality of the plasma is increased by the intravenous injection of hypertonic solutions such as mannitol or urea, there is a delay of up to several hours in the rise of osmolality of the CSF.

ii. It is during this period that the hyperosmolality of the blood dehydrates the brain and decreases the volume of CSF.

41. What is Queckenstedt test?

Ans. In the absence of subarachnoid block, compression of jugular vein, there is a rapid rise in pressure of 100 to 200 mm of water and a return to its original level within a few seconds after release.

42. What is Tobey-Ayer test?

Ans. Failure of pressure to rise with compression of one jugular vein but not the other may indicate lateral sinus thrombosis.

43. What is blood–brain barrier?

Ans. i. It is formed by endothelium of the choroidal and brain capillaries.

ii. Plasma membrane and adventitia of these vessels.

iii. Pericapillary foot process of the astrocytes.

44. Are there lymphatic channels in the nervous system?

Ans. i. No.

ii. Since the brain and spinal cord have no lymphatic channels, the CSF through its sink action serves to remove the waste products of cerebral metabolism, the main ones being carbon dioxide, lactate or hydrogen ions.

45. What is the intracranial volume?

Ans.

Volume of the brain	:	1400 ml
CSF volume	:	150 ml
Blood volume	:	150 ml
Average intracranial volume	:	1700 ml

46. How much is CSF formed every day?

Ans. i. The CSF is formed at approximately 500 ml/day or 0.3 ml/minute.

ii. The CSF as a whole is therefore renewed four or five times daily.

47. Discuss the circulation of CSF.

Ans. a. From its principal site of formation in the choroid plexus of the lateral ventricle.

b. The CSF flows downward through the third ventricle, aqueduct, fourth ventricle and foramen of magenda (medially) and lushka (laterally) at the base of the medulla to the perimedullary and peripheral subarachnoid space.

c. Then around the brain stem and rostrally to the basal and ambient cisterns, through the tentorial aperature and finally to the lateral and superior surface of the cerebral hemispheres where most of it is absorbed.

48. Discuss CSF absorption.

Ans. i. Absorption of CSF is through arachnoid villi.

ii. CSF and ICP pressures which are in equilibrium are derived largely from the transmitted vascular pressure and not from CSF outflow resistance.

However, in pathological states such as bacterial meningitis and subarachnoid haemorrhage, the resistance may rise to levels that impede CSF circulation and cause hydrocephalus.

49. What is transmantle pressure?

Ans. The pressure difference between the ventricles and the subarachnoid space is transmantle pressure.

50. What is the correlation of carbon dioxide and CSF?

Ans. i. The retention or inhalation of carbon dioxide raises the blood PCO_2 and correspondingly decreases the PH of CSF. This acidification of CSF acts as a potent cerebral vasodilator causing an increase in cerebral blood flow and leads to intracranial hypertension.

ii. Hyperventilation which reduces PCO_2 has the opposite effect. It increases the PH and the cerebral vascular resistance and thereby decreasing CSF pressure. The maneuver of lowering the arterial CO_2 content by hyperventilation is utilized in the treatment of acutely raised ICP.

51. What is Monro-Kellie doctrine?

Ans. i. The intact cranium forms a rigid container such that an increase in any one of its contents—brain, blood, CSF will elevate the ICP.

ii. According to Monro-Kellie doctrine, an increase in volume of any of these three components must be at the expense of the other two.

52. What are the changes that take place when there is a raised ICP?

Ans. i. Displacement of CSF from cranial cavity into the spinal canal.

ii. Stretching of dura (falx cerebri and tentorium cerebelli and deformation of the brain.

53. What is intracranial compliance?

Ans. i. The change in ICP for a given change in intracranial volume.

ii. Normal is 2 to 5 mmHg.

iii. The normal compliance curve begins its steep accent at an ICP of approximately 25 mmHg after these small increases in intracranial volume results in marked elevation of ICP.

iv. ICP elevation results in

a. Herniation of the brain

b. Reduces the volume of intracranial blood contained in the veins and dural sinuses.

54. What is cerebral perfusion pressure (CPP)?

Ans.
i. CPP is defined as the mean systemic arterial (MAP) minus the ICP that provides the driving force for circulation across the capillary bed of the brain.

$$CPP = MAP - ICP$$

It is the numerical difference between ICP and mean blood pressure within the ventricle.

ii. Elevation of ICP that approximates the level of mean systemic blood pressure eventually causes a widespread reduction in cerebral blood flow and perfusion and can cause ischaemia and brain death.

iii. The
a. Severity and
b. Duration of reduced CPP are the main determinants of cerebral damage.

iv. A high ICP and a low BP may combine to reduce cerebral perfusion pressure and cause diffuse ischaemic damage.

v. Cerebral blood flow (CBF) increases with hypercapnia and acidosis and decreases with hypocapnia and alkalosis. This forms the basis for the use of hyperventilation to lower the ICP and this effect on ICP is mediated through a decrease in intracranial blood volume.

55. What is autoregulation?

Ans.
i. Refers to physiologic response whereby cerebral blood flow (CBF) remains relatively constant over a wide range of blood pressure (50 mmHg to 150 mmHg) as a consequence of alteration of cerebrovascular resistance.

ii. If the systemic blood pressure drops, cerebral perfusion is preserved through vasodilatation of arterioles in the brain likewise arteriolar vasoconstriction occurs at high systemic pressure to prevent hyperperfusion.

iii. Perfusion is increased in sitting, hypoxic or hyper-ventilation.

56. What are the normal ICP and CPP parameters?

Ans.
i. ICP should be maintained at less than 20 mmHg.
ii. CPP should be maintained at more than 70 mmHg.

57. What is the vicious cycle in cerebral disorder?

Ans.   i. CPP = MAP–ICP.

   ii. Elevated ICP diminishes cerebral perfusion and can lead to tissue ischaemia.

   iii. Ischaemia may in turn lead to vasodilatation via auto-regulatory mechanisms designed to restore cerebral perfusion (therefore treat ischaemia with vasopressors).

   iv. However, vasodilatation also increases cerebral blood volume which in turn increases ICP that lowers CPP and provokes further ischaemia.

   v. The vicious cycle is commonly seen in:

     a. Traumatic brain injury

     b. Massive intracerebral haemorrhage

     c. Large hemispheric infarct with significant tissue shift.

58. Discuss the treatment of hyperventilation in raise ICP.

Ans.   i. Emergent treatment of elevated ICP is most quickly achieved by intubation and hyperventilation which causes vasoconstriction and reduced cerebral blood volume.

   ii. Because of the concern of provoking cerebral ischaemia hyperventilation is used for short period of time until a more definitive treatment can be instituted.

   iii. Furthermore, the effects of continued hyperventilation on ICP are shortlived, often only for several hours because of the buffering capacity of the cerebral interstitium and rebound elevated ICP may accompany discontinuation of hyperventilation.

59. Describe brain edema.

Ans.   Brian edema is dangerous as it leads to increased intracranial pressure. It is of two types:

   1. *Vasogenic edema*:

     a. Vasogenic edema refers to the influx of the fluid and solute into the brain through an incompetent BBB. Typically vasogenic edema develops rapidly following injury.

b. It is due to compromise of BBB. In the normal cerebral vasculature, endothelial type junctions associated with astrocytes create an impermeable membrane (BBB) through which access into the brain interstitium is dependent upon specific transport mechanisms.

c. BBB may be compromised in ischaemia, trauma, infection and metabolic derangement.

2. *Cytotoxic edema*:

a. It refers to cellular swelling and occurs in a variety of settings including brain ischaemia and trauma.

b. Early astrocytic swelling is a hallmark of ischaemia.

60. What is ischaemic penumbra?

Ans. i. It refers to ischaemic brain tissue that has not yet undergone irreversible infarction implying that the region is potentially salvageable if ischaemia can be reversed.

ii. Hypoxemia triggers the pathogenic mechanisms by causing calcium influx.

61. What are secondary brain insults?

Ans. i. Factors that may exacerbate ischaemic brain injury including systemic hypotension, hypoxia which further reduce substrate delivery to vulnerable brain tissue.

ii. Fever, seizures, hyperglycemia which can increase cellular metabolism outstripping compensatory processes.

iii. Clinically these events are known as secondary brain events because they lead to exacerbation of the primary brain injury.

62. What is apoptosis?

Ans. Apoptosis is programmed cell death.

63. What is histotoxic hypoxia?

Ans. i. Carbon monoxide

ii. Cyanide poisoning are termed as histotoxic hypoxia since they cause a direct impairment of the respiratory chain.

64. What is the triad of Wernicke's disease?

Ans. It is a triad of:

   i. Ophthalmoplegia

   ii. Ataxia

   iii. Global confusion.

65. Describe hypoxic encephalopathy.

Ans. i. If circulation is restored within 3 to 5 minutes, full recovery may occur, but if hypoxic – ischaemic bouts persist beyond 3 to 5 minutes, some degrees of persistent cerebral damage is the rule.

   ii. The hippocampus CA neurons are vulnerable to even brief episodes of hypoxic – ischaemia perhaps explaining why isolated persistent memory deficits may occur after brief cardiac arrest.

   iii. A specific form of hypoxic – ischaemic encephalopathy so called watershed infarcts occurs in the distal territories between the major cerebral arteries and can cause cognitive deficits including visual agnosia and weakness is greater in proximal than in distal muscle groups.

   iv. *Diagnosis*:

      • BP less than 70 mmHg

      • $PaCO_2$ less than 40 mmHg.

   v. *Treatment*:

      • Post-hypoxic myoclonus

        – Clonazepam 1.5 to 10 mg

        – Sodium valproate 300 to 1200 mg.

66. What are the causes of raised ICP?

Ans. a. A cerebral or extradural mass (e.g. SDH)

   b. Generalised brain swelling (e.g. ischaemic anoxic states)

   c. An increase in venous pressure (e.g. SSS thrombosis)

   d. Obstruction to the flow and absorption of CSF (meningitis)

   e. Any process that expands the volume of CSF (e.g. choroid plexus tumour: Increases CSF production).

67. **What are the clinical features of raised ICP?**

Ans.   i. Headache

   ii. Nausea and vomiting

   iii. Drowsiness (only when ICP exceeds 40 to 50 mmHg) enables cerebral perfusion (CPP) and cerebral blood flow diminish to a degree that results in loss of consciousness

   iv. Ocular palsies

   v. *Pupillary dilatation*: Generally corresponds to an ICP of 28 to 34 mmHg

   vi. *Papilledema*: Optic atrophy, blindness

   vii. *In children*: Enlargement of head because cranial sutures have not closed.

68. **What is hydrocephalus ex vacuo or colpocephaly?**

Ans.   It is a ventricular enlargement due to failure of development of brain.

69. **What is Dandy-Walker syndrome?**

Ans.   It is a congenital failure of opening of foramina.

70. **What is the correlation of obstruction to ventricular enlargement?**

Ans.   Ventricle closest to the obstruction enlarges the most.

71. **What are the radiological features of external hydrocephalus?**

Ans.   The radiological features of enlarged subarachnoid space over and between the cerebral hemispheres coupled with modest enlargement of the lateral ventricle, e.g. subdural hygroma, arachnoid cysts.

72. **What is acute hydrocephalus?**

Ans.   Processes such as subarachnoid haemorrhage and cerebral haemorrhage or brain abscess that ruptures into the ventricle and rapidly expands the volume of CSF.

73. **What are the clinical varieties of hydrocephalus?**

Ans.   i. *Overt tension hydrocephalus*: This occurs very early in life and causes enlargement of the head.

ii. *Occult hydrocephalus*: In it, the hydrocephalus becomes symptomatic after the cranial sutures have fused and the head remains normal in size.

iii. *Normal pressure hydrocephalus*: An occult hydrocephalus is arrested or compensated hydrocephalus of late adult life.

iv. Acute hydrocephalus.

74. What is infantile hydrocephalus or overt congenital hydrocephalus?

Ans. i. The cranial bones fuse by the end of third year.

ii. *Diastasis*: Marked increase of ICP, particularly if it evolves rapidly may separate the newly formed sutures.

iii. Usual causes:
- Intraventricular matrix haemorrhage in premature infants
- Fetal and neonatal infections
- Type II chiari malformations
- Aqueductal atresia and stenosis
- Dandy-Walker syndrome.

75. What are the causes of acute hydrocephalus?

Ans. i. SAH (subarachnoid haemorrhage)

ii. AVM (arterio-venous malformation)

iii. Deep hemispherical haemorrhage that dissects into ventricle

iv. Fourth ventricular obstruction by tumour/cerebellar-brain stem haemorrhage.

76. What are the neuropathologic effects of tension hydrocephalus?

Ans. i. Ventricular expansion tends to be maximal in frontal horns and hence frontal lobe, basal ganglionic – frontal motor activity are affected.

ii. Transependymal movement of water.

77. What is normal pressure hydrocephalus?

Ans. i. Formation of CSF equilibrates with absorption.

ii. Triad of clinical features:
  • Gait disorder
  • Impairment of mental function
  • Sphincter disturbance
iii. CSF pressure is usually above 155 mm of water.

78. What is slit-ventricle syndrome?

Ans. i. The appearance of ventricle on imaging is slit like.
  ii. It is a complication of shunting seen in children.
  iii. These patients develop a low-pressure syndrome with severe generalized headache often with nausea and vomiting whenever they sit up or stand.
  iv. *Treatment*: To replace the shunt valve with another that opens under or higher pressure would suffice.

79. What is the treatment of NPH?

Ans. Acetazolamide (inhibits CSF production): 250 to 500 mg.

80. What is otic hydrocephalus?

Ans. Lateral sinus thrombosis due to venous obstruction causing a raised intracranial pressure.

81. What is regional arachnoiditis?

Ans. Limited to lumbosacral roots
Causes:
  • Ruptured disc
  • Myelogram
  • Spinal surgery
  • Chemically contaminated spinal anesthetics.

82. What causes opticochiasmatic arachnoiditis and pachymeningitis?

Ans. Neurosyphilis.

83. What are idiopathic intracranial hypertension and pseudotumour cerebri?

Ans. i. There are due to functional obstruction to outflow in the venous sinuses.

ii. Elevated spinal fluid pressure has been attributed to a blockage of CSF absorption by proteinaceous fluid, e.g. GBS

iii. Increased ICP (250 to 450 mm of water)

iv. Seen usually in overweight women with menstrual irregularities

v. Use of oral contraceptives

vi. The diagnosis of idiopathic pseudotumour cerebri should not be accepted when the content of CSF is abnormal

vii. Visual loss

viii. *Treatment*:
- Weight reduction, steroids
- Shunting, optic nerve sheath fenestration.

83. What is intracranial hypotension?

Ans. i. May be seen as lumbar puncture headache

ii. Spontaneous intracranial hypotension
- No cause
- After straining

iii. Prominent dural enhancement with gadolinium of MRI due to dural venous dilatation.

84. What causes hemosiderosis?

Ans. i. Repeated contamination of meninges by blood

ii. Oozing vascular malformation

iii. Tumour.

85. What infections cause ependymal involvement?

Ans. i. Mumps

ii. Toxoplasmosis

iii. Tumour (craniopharingioma).

26

Coma and Brain Death

1. What is consciousness?

Ans. It is the state of awareness of self and environment and responsiveness to external stimulation and inner need.

2. What is coma?

Ans. a. The patient who appears to be asleep and is at the same time incapable of being aroused by external stimuli or inner need is in a state of coma.

b. State of arousal, content of consciousness are the components of coma.

c. Two-thirds of causes of coma are metabolic and one-third are due to structural.

d. Cardiac arrest with cerebral hypoperfusion and head injuries are the most common causes of the vegetative and minimally conscious states.

3. Discuss the anatomy and physiology of coma.

Ans. The diminished alertness is due to widespread abnormalities of the cerebral hemispheres or due to reduced activity of a special thalamocortical alerting system—the reticular activating system.

Therefore, the important causes of coma are:

• Lesions that damage the RAS or its projections

• Destruction of large portions of both cerebral hemispheres

• Suppression of reticulocerebral function by drugs, toxins or metabolic derangements such as hypoglycemia, anoxia, uremia and hepatic failure.

4. Discuss the metabolic disorders causing coma.

Ans. Systemic metabolic abnormalities cause coma by:
- Interrupting the delivery of energy substrates (hypoxia, ischaemia, hypoglycemia).
- By altering neuronal excitability (drug and alcohol intoxication, anesthesia and epilepsy.
- In all these metabolic encephalopathies, the degree of neurologic change depends to a large extent on the rapidity with which the serum changes occur.
- In a drowsy and confused patient, bilateral *asterixis* is a certain sign of metabolic encephalopathy or drug intoxication.
- Normal pupillary size and light reaction distinguishes most drug induced comas from structural brain stem damage.

5. Correlate serum sodium levels with the states of reduced alertness.

Ans. i. Sodium levels less than 125 mmol/L induce confusion.
ii. Sodium levels less than 115 mmol/L are associated with coma and convulsions.

6. Discuss epileptic coma.

Ans. The self-limited coma that follows seizures is termed as the postictal state. It may be due to exhaustion of energy reserves or effects of locally toxic molecules that are the by-products of seizures.

7. Discuss the metabolic parameters of cerebral neurons.

Ans. Cerebral neurons are fully dependent on cerebral blood flow (CBF) and the related delivery of oxygen and glucose.
- CBF is 75 ml/100 g/min in gray matter and 30 ml/per 100 g/min in white matter.
- Oxygen consumption is 3.5 ml/100 g/min.
- Glucose utilization is 5 mg/100/min.
- Brain stores of glucose provide energy for 2 min after blood flow is interrupted.

- Oxygen stores last 8–10 seconds after the cessation of blood flow.
- Simultaneous hypoxia and ischaemia exhaust glucose more rapidly.

8. Discuss the structural causes of coma due to space occupying lesions including herniation.

Ans. i. Herniation refers to displacement of brain tissue into a compartment that it normally does not occupy.

ii. The clinical signs are either due to the mass itself or false localizing signs.

iii. False localizing signs are due to compression of brain structures at a distance from the mass.
Duret haemorrhage: Secondary brain stem haemorrhage due to trauma.

iv. Types of cerebral herniation are:
- Uncal
- Central
- Transfacial
- Foraminal.

v. *The Kernohan-Woltman sign*: In some cases, the lateral displacement of the midbrain due to uncal transtentorial herniation causes compression of the opposite cerebral peduncle, producing a Babinski sign and hemiparesis contralateral to the original hemiparesis.

vi. In cases of acutely appearing masses, horizontal displacement of the pineal calcification of 3–5 mm is generally associated with drowsiness, 6–8 mm with stupor and more than 9 mm with coma.

9. What are decorticate rigidity and decerebrate rigidity and what do they suggest?

Ans. *Decortication*: Flexion of the elbows and wrists and supination of the arm. It suggests bilateral damage rostral to the midbrain.
Decerebration: Extension of the elbows and wrists with pronation. It indicates damage to the motor tracts in the midbrain or caudal diencephalon.

10. Discuss pupillary signs in coma.

Ans.   i. Normally reactive and round pupils of midsize (2.5 to 5 mm) essentially exclude midbrain damage, either primary or secondary to compression.

ii. One unreactive and enlarged pupil (more than 6 mm) or one that is poorly reactive signifies compression of the third nerve from the effects of a mass above.

iii. The most extreme pupillary sign, bilaterally dilated and unreactive pupils, indicates severe midbrain damage usually from compression by a supratentorial mass.

iv. Unilateral miosis in coma has been attributed to dysfunction of sympathetic efferents originating in the posterior hypothalamus and descending in the tegmentum of the brain stem to the cervical cord.

v. Very small but reactive pupils (less than 1 mm) characterize narcotic or barbiturate overdoses but also occur with extensive pontine haemorrhage.

11. Explain the maxim: "the eyes look toward a hemispheral lesion and away from a brain stem lesion".

Ans.   i. Frontal eye field area number eight stimulates the movement of eyes towards the opposite side (as a phenomenon of saccades). Hence, when a frontal hemispheral lesion is present, the opposite intact frontal hemisphere pushes the eyes towards the affected hemisphere and therefore the maxim "the eyes look toward a hemispheral lesion."

ii. The supranuclear pathways subserving saccadic horizontal gaze to the LEFT—the pathway originates in the right frontal cortex, descends in the internal.

Capsule decussates at the level of the rostral pons and descends to synapse in the left pontine paramedian reticular formation (PPRF).

Therefore, in a brain stem (pons) since the tract has already crossed, the maxim "the eyes look away from a brain stem lesion."

12. What is ocular bobbing?

Ans. Ocular bobbing describes brisk downward and slow upward movements of eyes associated with loss of horizontal eye movements and is diagnostic of bilateral pontine damage usually from a thrombosis of the basilar artery.

13. What is ocular dipping?

Ans. Ocular dipping is a slower arrhythmic downward movement followed by a faster upward movement in patients with normal reflex horizontal gaze. It indicates diffuse cortical anoxic damage.

14. Discuss oculocephalic reflexes (doll's eye movement).

Ans.
i. The oculocephalic reflexes depend on the integrity of the ocular motor nuclei and their interconnecting tracts that extend from the midbrain to the pons and medulla.
ii. These reflexes are elicited by moving the head from side to side or vertically and observing evoked eye movements in the direction opposite to the head movement.
iii. These movements are normally suppressed in the awake patient.
iv. The ability to elicit them therefore indicated a reduced cortical influence on the brain stem.
v. Preservation of evoked reflex eye movements signifies the integrity of the brain stem and implies that the origin of unconsciousness lies in the cerebral hemispheres.
vi. The opposite, an absence of reflex eye movements, usually signify damage within the brain stem.

15. Discuss oculovestibular response.

Ans.
i. The test is performed by irrigating the external auditory canal with cool water in order to induce convection currents in the labyrinths.
ii. After a brief latency, the result is tonic deviation of both eyes to the side of cool-water irrigation and nystagmus in the opposite direction (cows—cold water opposite warm water same).

iii. The loss of conjugate ocular movements indicates brain stem damage.

iv. The absence of nystagmus despite conjugate deviation of the globes indicates that the cerebral hemispheres are damaged or metabolically suppressed.

16. Discuss corneal reflex.

Ans. i. By touching the cornea with a wisp of cotton, a response consisting of brief bilateral lid closure is normally observed.

ii. The corneal reflexes depend on the integrity of pontine pathways between the fifth (afferent) and both seventh (efferent) cranial nerves.

iii. They are important clinical tests of pontine function.

17. Discuss the respiratory patterns in coma.

Ans. i. *Cheyne-Stokes respiration:*
- This phenomenon has been attributed to isolation of the brain stem respiratory centers from the cerebrum, rendering them more sensitive than usual to carbon dioxide.
- It is postulated that as a result of overbreathing, the blood carbon dioxide drops below the concentration required to stimulate the centers and breathing gradually stops.
- Carbon dioxide then reaccumulates until it exceeds the respiratory threshold and the cycle then repeats itself.
- Alternatively, the periodicity has been attributed to the stimulating effect of a low arterial PO_2 depressed respiratory center.
- In either case, the presence of Cheyne-Stokes breathing signifies bilateral dysfunction of cerebral structures.

ii. *Central neurogenic hyperventilation (CNH):*
- Lesions of the lower midbrain—upper pontine tegmentum, may give rise to CNH.
- This disorder is characterized by an increase in the rate and depth of respiration to an extent that produces advanced respiratory alkalosis.

iii. *Apneustic breathing*:
- Low pontine lesions cause apneustic breathing.
- In this, a few rapid deep breaths alternate with apneic cycles.

iv. *Biot breathing (ataxia of breathing)*:
- It is seen in the lesions of the dorsomedial part of the medulla.
- The rhythm of breathing is chaotic, being irregularly interrupted and each breath varying in rate and depth.

Summary:
- One may observe a succession of respiratory patterns.
- Then Cheyne-Stokes
- Then CNH
  - Then apneustic breathing
  - Biot breathing
  - Indicating an extension of the functional disorder from upper to lower brain stem.

18. Summarise the brain stem reflexes in coma?

Ans. Examination of brainstem reflexes in coma:
- Midbrain and third nerve function are tested by pupillary reaction to light.
- Pontine function by spontaneous and reflex eye movements and corneal responses.
- Medullary function by respiratory and pharyngeal responses.

19. Discuss the usefulness of EEG in coma.

Ans. i. The amount of background slowing of the EEG is a reflection of the severity of any diffuse encephalopathy.

ii. Predominant high-voltage slowing (triphasic waves) in the frontal region is typical of metabolic coma as from hepatic failure.

iii. Widespread fast (δ) activity implicates sedative drugs (diazepines, barbiturates).

iv. *Alpha coma*: A special pattern, it is defined by widespread variable 8–12 hertz activity, superficially resembles the normal α rhythm of waking but is unresponsive to environmental stimuli. It results from pontine or diffuse cortical damage and is associated with a poor prognosis.

v. EEG recordings may reveal clinically in apparent epileptic discharges in a patient with coma.

vi. Normal α activity on the EEG which is suppressed by stimulating the patient also alerts the clinician to the locked-in syndrome, hysteria.

20. Discuss the differential diagnosis of coma.

Ans. i. Diseases that cause no focal or lateralizing neurologic signs usually with normal brain stem functions, CT scan and cellular content of the CSF are normal.

Examples:
- Intoxications
- Metabolic disturbances
- Post-seizure states

ii. Diseases that cause meningeal irritation with or without fever and with an excess of WBCs or RBCs in the CSF, usually without focal or lateralizing cerebral or brain stem signs, CT or MRI shows no mass lesion.

Examples:
- Subarachnoid haemorrhage
- Meningitis

iii. Diseases that cause focal brain stem or lateralizing cerebral signs with or without changes in CSF, CT and MRI are abnormal.

Examples:
- Stroke
- Tumour
- Brain abscess.

21. What are the treatable causes of coma?

Ans. i. Drug and alcohol intoxication
ii. Infections
iii. Epidural and subdural haematoma
iv. Brain abscess

v. Meningitis

vi. Status epilepticus

vii. Metabolic coma (*Examples*: Hypoglycemia, hyponatremia).

22. Discuss brain death.

Ans. This is a state of cessation of cerebal function while somatic function is maintained by artificial means and the heart continues to pump.

They contain three essential elements of clinical evidence.

i. Widespread cortical destruction that is reflected by deep coma and unresponsiveness to all forms of stimulation.

ii. Global brain stem damage demonstrated by absent pupillary light reaction and by the loss of occulovestibular and corneal reflexes.

iii. Destruction of the medulla manifested by complete apnea.

The pulse rate is invariant and unresponsive to atropine.

Apnea test is used to confirm brain death.

Index